LECTURE NOTES ON
OCCUPATIONAL MEDICINE

H.A. WALDRON
TUC Centenary Institute of Occupational Health,
London School of Hygiene and Tropical Medicine,
London, WC1E 7HT

THIRD EDITION

BLACKWELL SCIENTIFIC PUBLICATIONS

OXFORD LONDON EDINBURGH

BOSTON PALO ALTO MELBOURNE

© 1976, 1979, 1985 by
Blackwell Scientific Publications
Editorial offices:
Osney Mead, Oxford, OX2 0EL
8 John Street, London, WC1N 2ES
23 Ainslie Place, Edinburgh, EH3 6AJ
52 Beacon Street, Boston
  Massachusetts 02108, USA
744 Cowper Street, Palo Alto
  California 94301, USA
107 Barry Street, Carlton
  Victoria 3053, Australia

First published 1976
Reprinted 1977
Second edition 1979
Third edition 1985

Set by Enset (Photosetting)
Midsomer Norton, Bath, Avon
and printed and bound
in Great Britain by
Butler & Tanner Ltd
Frome and London

DISTRIBUTORS

USA
  Blackwell Mosby Book Distributors
  11830 Westline Industrial Drive
  St Louis, Missouri 63141

Canada
  Blackwell Mosby Book Distributors
  120 Melford Drive, Scarborough
  Ontario, M1B 2X4

Australia
  Blackwell Scientific Book Distributors
  31 Advantage Road, Highett
  Victoria 3190

British Library
Cataloguing in Publication Data

Waldron, H.A.
  Lecture notes on occupational
  medicine.—3rd ed.
  1. Medicine, Industrial
  I. Title
  616.9'803   RC963

  ISBN 0-632-01198-X

CONTENTS

PREFACE TO THIRD EDITION

The success of this little book provides me with a constant source of pleasure and surprise; it also enables me, in this new edition, to take account of the helpful suggestions which some of its readers have made and to correct some of the mistakes which they have taken the trouble to point out to me. To all these volunteer proofreaders I express my gratitude.

In the present edition I have expanded the section on the toxicology of industrial poisons even though, as I say several times in the text, the prevalence of the toxic industrial diseases is on the decline in the fully industrialized countries. There are several reasons for this apparent anomaly; first, there is a considerable amount of recent work which needs to be mentioned; second, it is still my belief that the practice of occupational medicine has to be founded on a good knowledge of toxicology since it is impossible to give an opinion on any of the presumed effects of a toxic substance without a sound working knowledge of its metabolism and toxicology and finally, the toxic diseases are still common in the developing countries and it is my hope that this book will be helpful to practitioners in those countries.

A book of this nature cannot but reflect the particular interests and prejudices of its author and I make no pretence that it is sufficient for a complete understanding of occupational medicine. I hope that those who read it, however, will find it a useful introduction to the subject and that it will stimulate them to wish to learn more about it. To the students who use it, I send my best wishes for their success in the examination game and I apologize in advance if anything I have said here leads them into error.

PREFACE TO FIRST EDITION

The relationship between occupation and health has been recognized for several hundred years, but it is a topic which is still generally under-represented in the medical curriculum. This book presents to the medical student a concise view of the subject in a way which I hope will stimulate him to take more account of the occupation of those patients whom he will see, both in his training and, later, in his professional life. I have particularly stressed the interaction between occupational medicine and other areas of environmental health and suggested that hazards which arise from certain industrial processes are a risk, not merely to those within the walls of the factories in which they are carried out.

There are many excellent texts for the specialist in occupational medicine and I would not expect him to find much here which he did not already know. Others whose field of interest is not primarily with occupational health may find it useful, however, especially those whose work in general practice frequently brings them into contact with illnesses which may have their origins wholly or in part, in their patient's work.

CHAPTER 1/THE EFFECTS OF
OCCUPATION ON HEALTH

✗ The knowledge that man's health can be intimately connected with his occupation must have become apparent at an early stage of social evolution. The first occupational disease was probably silicosis occurring in the makers of flint tools. Excavations of stone-age sites suggest that the manufacture of flint tools was a specialized occupation and hut floors covered by thousands of pieces of flint debris leave no doubt that the tool makers were heavily exposed to silica. The next most ancient occupational disease might have been farmer's lung which followed the domestication of grain. In general, however, the prevalence of occupational disease would have been low before the introduction of metal working and mining. The ancient physicians, who were extremely acute observers and who recognized that other environmental factors could promote ill health, tended to ignore the effects of occupation. This may have been because the more onerous tasks were undertaken by slaves or prisoners—the lead mines of antiquity were worked by slave labour, for example, and exacted a heavy loss of life—thus placing them beyond the care of the physician. Some texts on the disease of miners appeared during the fifteenth and sixteenth centuries, but no comprehensive treatise on occupational medicine was produced before 1700 when Ramazzini published *De Morbis Artificum*. The modern development of the subject of occupational medicine can be traced directly from Ramazzini's book. His own interest had its origins in a singularly unglamorous event, as he explains:

> The Accident, from which I took occasion to write this Treatise of the Diseases of Tradesmen is as follows. In this City, which is very populous for its Bigness, and is built both close and high, it is usual to have their Houses of Office (cesspits) cleansed every third Year; and, while the Men employed in this Work were cleansing that at my House, I took notice of one of them, who worked with a great deal of Anxiety and Eagerness, and, being moved with Compassion I asked the poor Fellow, Why he did not work more calmly and avoid over-tiring himself with too much Straining? Upon this the poor Wretch lifted up his Eyes from the dismal Vault, and replied, That none but those who have tried it could imagine the Trouble of

staying above four Hours in that Place, it being equally troublesome as to be struck blind. After he came out of the Place, I took a
narrow View of his Eyes, and found them very red and dim; upon
which I asked him, If they had any usual Remedy of that Disorder?
He replied, their only Way was to run immediately Home, and
confine themselves for a Day to a dark Room, and wash their Eyes
now and then with warm Water; by which Means they used to find
their Pain somewhat assuaged. Then I asked him, if he felt any
Heat in his Throat, and Difficulty of Respiration, or Headache?
And whether the Smell affected their Nose, or occasioned a
Squeamishness? He answered, That he felt none of those
Inconveniences; that the only Parts which suffered were the Eyes,
and that if he continued longer at the same Work, without
Interruption, he should be blind in a short Time, as it had
happened to others. Immediately after he clapt his Hands over his
Eyes, and run Home. After this I took notice of several Beggars in
the City, who, having been employed in that Work, were either very
weak-sighted, or absolutely blind.

Ramazzini it was who suggested that in addition to the questions
recommended by Hippocrates, the physician should ask the patient one
more, namely what is your occupation? This piece of advice has yet to
become properly implemented!

The Industrial Revolution produced an upheaval in the social life of
this country the repercussions of which are still being felt. Industry
sprawled over the countryside at will, tending to concentrate in the areas
where there were readily available sources of energy and raw materials,
and in the wake of industry came the squalid towns, hastily built to house
the new urban work force. The conditions in the factories and the mines
were terrible and resulted in great morbidity and mortality, which in turn
had serious economic consequences. During the nineteenth century a
series of Acts was passed through Parliament which resulted in a gradual
improvement in the lot of the working population. In the beginning, the
motivation behind these apparently philanthropic efforts was dictated by
the desire of the mill owners to improve efficiency; a sick or dying
employee could not work as well as one in reasonable health and was
thus uneconomic. To improve the conditions of the workers was, therefore, necessary to ensure the greatest return on capital.

The first Act which related to working conditions was the Health and
Morals of Apprentices Act passed in the reign of George III in 1802.
This Act stipulated that children in the cotton and woollen mills should
work no more than a maximum of 12 hours a day, should do no night

work and that their places of work should be ventilated and washed down twice a year! The Act fixed no minimum age for the employment of children. The 1819 Act for the Regulation of Cotton Mills and Factories attempted to remedy this omission by fixing the minimum age of employment at 9, but this Act, like the 1802 Act failed from the want of an effective mechanism to enforce its provisions. To overcome this defect, another Act was passed in 1825 which required every mill owner to enter into a book the name of any child in his employ who appeared to be under the age of 9, together with the names of its parents. It was then incumbent upon the parents to sign a document stating that the child *was* over the legal age, thus absolving the mill owner from any blame in the event of subsequent legal proceedings. This somewhat inept law invited abuse so that yet another Act was required to close this loophole. Under the provisions of the Act of 1833 each employed child was required to have a medical certificate stating that it was of the appearance and ordinary strength of a child of 9. This Act was of course as open to abuse as its predecessor but it had the important effect of bringing the medical profession directly into the administration of factory legislation. And what was of greater significance, it established the Factory Inspectorate. The Medical Branch of the Factory Inspectorate was not introduced at this time and it was 1898 before it came into being.

As the nineteenth century progressed many more Acts were passed, designed to improve the conditions of employment and, little by little, conditions for the working population did improve. Improvement is a relative term, however, and many dreadful practices flourished well towards the end of the century; boys were still put up chimneys until 1875, for example, and accounts of the pitiful privations suffered by the working class are to be found in many Victorian novels. Occupational diseases were common and were accepted as the normal consequence of being employed. Many of the occupational diseases were known by colloquial names, a number of which have survived into our own time. This is some indication both that they were common, and of such a gross character that the general public was able to recognize and classify their symptoms.

There is no gainsaying the fact that compared with a generation or two ago, the conditions under which the mass of the population works have improved beyond measure. Largely because of this, doctors have tended to lose sight of the pathogenicity of occupation unless they are confronted with one of the classical industrial diseases, and it is still with these that the major part of occupational medicine is concerned. It is becoming increasingly evident, however, that environmental factors are amongst the major determinants of health. For most men, the environment which has the greatest effect upon their health is to be found at their place of work. About one-third of a man's life is spent at work and a lesser, but still substantial proportion of that of many women. For these reasons alone no practitioner, whatever his speciality can afford to overlook his patients' job.

Many occupations do appear to carry with them an increased risk of mortality, as reference to Table 1.1, which shows the 20 occupations with the highest SMR*, makes clear. It is not difficult to reconcile some occupations with high SMRs; fishing, steel erecting and coal mining are inherently sufficiently dangerous that it comes as no surprise that the lives of their practitioners may be in jeopardy. The factors which might account for the increased risks amongst electrical engineers, shoe makers and watch repairers are not so immediately obvious, however. Publicans, on the other hand, have been recognized for many years to be following an occupation likely to shorten their lives. William Farr, the first medical commentator in the Registrar General's office wrote in 1861 that the publican has only to abstain from excesses in spirits and other strong drinks to live as long as other people. Farr exemplifies here the British characteristic of disapproving of those who provide them with their pleasures!

On a more happy note, there are also a number of occupations which carry with them a decreased mortality and the 20 with the lowest SMRs are listed in Table 1.2. On the whole the list is dominated by those in the professions; the low SMR enjoyed by university teachers is especially gratifying. That Ministers of the Crown and senior government officials are also unduly hearty puts the lie to their frequently expressed belief that theirs is a life of constant stress and toil; if it is, then it certainly does not adversely affect their chances of living to enjoy their pensions.

When interpreting SMRs, however, a number of factors must be borne in mind. One of the most important is to separate out the effects due to occupation from those due to social class (see Table 1.3). One way in which this can be done is by relating the mortality of the men in an occupational group to that of their wives, the wives being used as a control for socio-economic factors.

*SMR = Standardized mortality ratio. It is the ratio of the observed number of deaths amongst an occupational group compared with the number which would have been expected had the mortality rates of the population at large been experienced, allowing for age correction, i.e. SMR = observed deaths/expected deaths × 100. An SMR greater than 100 indicates that the group under consideration has a greater than usual mortality whilst the converse is true if the SMR is less than 100.

Table 1.1. Twenty occupations with the highest SMRs*

Occupation	SMR
Electrical engineers, so described	317
Bricklayers', etc., labourers, nec	273
Deck and engineroom ratings, barge and boatmen	233
Deck, engineering officers and ship pilots	175
Fishermen	171
Steel erectors; riggers	164
Labourers and unskilled workers nec foundries in engineering and allied trade	160
Coal mine workers above ground	160
Shoemakers and shoe repairers	156
Machine tool operators	156
Publicans, innkeepers	155
Watch and chronometer makers and repairers	154
Leather product makers nec	147
Electronic engineers	145
Printers (so described)	144
Rolling, tube mill operators, metal drawers	144
Brewers, wine makers and related workers	143
Surface workers nec, mines and quarries	141
Coal mine workers underground	141

*From Registrar General's *Occupational Mortality Tables*, HMSO, 1978.

In many cases, the number of deaths within an occupational order may be small and then the SMR becomes misleading. It is necessary, therefore, to apply some statistical test to the SMR in order to determine whether the difference between the number of observed and expected deaths is due to factors other than chance. As a first approximation, and providing the number of deaths is large enough, the chi-squared statistic can be used where

$$\chi^2 = \frac{(\text{observed deaths} - \text{expected deaths})}{(\text{expected deaths})}.$$

Table 1.2. Twenty occupations with lowest SMR

Occupation	SMR
Trainee craftsmen (engineering and allied trades)	26
Electrical engineers	42
Labourers and unskilled workers nec coke ovens and gas works	46
Foremen (engineering and allied trades)	47
University teachers	49
Paper products makers	50
Technologist nec	52
Managers in building and contracting	54
Physiotherapists	55
Local authority senior officers	57
Teachers nec	57
Mechanical engineers	58
Technical and related workers nec	58
Typists, shorthand writers, secretaries	59
Company secretaries and registrars	60
Ministers of the Crown; MPs nec; senior government officials	61
Printing workers nec	62
Office managers nec	64
Public health inspectors	64
Office machine operators	65

*From Registrar General's *Occupational Mortality Tables*, HMSO, 1978.

Table 1.3. SMR by social class, men aged 15–64*

Social class	SMR
I	77
II	81
IIIN	99
IIIM	106
IV	114
V	137

*From Registrar General's *Occupational Mortality Tables*, HMSO, 1978.

Table 1.4. Occupational groups at special risk of dying from some categories of disease*

Disease category	Occupational groups	SMR
Infectious and parasitic diseases	Labourers, nec	206
	Miners and quarrymen	172
	Service, sport and recreation workers	136
Malignant neoplasms	Armed forces	161
	Furnace, forge, foundry and rolling mill workers	135
	Labourers, nec	133
	Construction workers	126
	Painters and decorators	123
Diseases of the nervous system	Miners and quarrymen	149
Diseases of the circulatory system	Armed forces	143
	Miners and quarrymen	137
	Textile workers	121
	Leather workers	120
Diseases of the respiratory system	Miners and quarrymen	244
	Labourers, nec	193
	Furnace, forge, foundry and rolling mill workers	167
	Glass and ceramic makers	163
	Leather workers	134
Diseases of the skin	Farmers, foresters and fishermen	208
	Paper and printing workers	167
	Painters and decorators	166
Diseases of the musculoskeletal system	Clothing workers	319

*From Registrar General's *Occupational Mortality Tables*, HMSO, 1978.

With one degree of freedom, a χ^2 value in excess of 3.84 signifies a 5 per cent probability that the differences between observed and expected numbers are due to chance.

Using this test, it is possible to show that some occupational groups are at a special risk of dying from certain categories of disease due to factors which are associated with their job (Table 1.4).

Another way in which SMRs may be unreliable is due to the introduction of selection factors which tend to bias the results. For example, men who are in poor health are unlikely to take up an occupation which is physically demanding. Similarly, men who develop a chronic disease will be likely to leave the job in which they became ill if it is taxing and enter a sedentary occupation or, alternatively drift into some unskilled labouring job. When a man's relatives are questioned as to his occupation after his death, they may well mention the last job which will duly be recorded even though it may not be the one in which the patient was subjected to the hazards which were responsible for his ill health (always supposing the job was of aetiological significance). Conversely, it may happen that the relatives of a dead man will refer back to what they see as a prestigious occupation even though he may not have followed it for many years. Widows of men who have ever been coal miners, for example, will often state that this was their husband's occupation even if he had been away from the pits for many years. This tendency, of course, may artificially enhance the apparent risks of some occupations. Thus it is of the greatest importance, when pursuing a proposed link between occupation and disease to record a full occupational history of the subjects in the group under study, having particular regard to length and time of exposure.

Finally, it must be remembered that the SMR is necessarily a relatively crude index, being composed of the total experience of the particular group to all causes of death. Thus it is possible to find within an occupational group some diseases which are more common than average even though the SMR for all causes may be insignificantly different from 100; it follows in these cases, that there are compensatory low SMRs for other causes of death which average out the overall death rate. For example, Table 1.5 shows 10 occupations in which a high SMR for bronchitis is found but in which the overall SMR is not greatly

Table 1.5. Occupations with a high SMR for bronchitis

Occupation	SMR Bronchitis	SMR All causes
Coal miners	1683	62
Glass and ceramic furnacemen	172	100
Rolling tube mill operators	168	104
Metal furnacemen	151	108
Plasterers	146	109
Bus conductors	138	105
Coal, gas and coke oven furnacemen	131	96
Brewers	131	103
Glass formers	130	95
Lorry drivers' mates	129	105

From Registrar General's *Occupational Mortality Tables*, HMSO, 1971.

increased. Some of these occupations clearly carry a risk of respiratory disease. It is really no surprise to find coal miners in their pre-eminent position. Others are unexpected—it is difficult to see how plastering and brewing might contribute to a risk from bronchitis, for example.

Morbidity

Occupational morbidity is less easy to study than mortality because death is an event which is readily quantified whereas morbidity is a much more subjective matter. Nevertheless, there are many studies which show that occupational groups do differ in their pattern of morbidity.

Absence from work

Absence from work due to certified sickness results in a staggering number of days of work lost by comparison with which, the time lost from other causes such as strikes is trivial.

There are a number of interesting features about sickness absence, very little of which is due to illness caused by the prescribed industrial diseases (Table 1.6). There are, for example, marked differences in the number of days lost according to age and region (Tables 1.6 and 1.7).

Table 1.6. Regional rates for days lost from work by males through certified sickness and prescribed diseases*

Region	Days lost/10^3 working population at risk	
	Certified sickness	Prescribed diseases
Northern	25 665	95
Yorkshire and Humberside	20 880	87
East Midlands	15 595	61
West Midlands	15 400	27
East Anglia	12 900	25
South East	11 100	16
South West	16 425	24
North West	21 815	44
Scotland	21 420	70
Wales	31 810	153
Mean	17 160	47

*Means for 5 years, 1968–1972. From *Digest of Statistics Analysing Certificates of Incapacity*, HMSO.

Table 1.7. Days lost from work by males through certified illness, by age group*

Age group years	Days lost/10^3 working population
< 20	6750
20–24	7700
25–29	8340
30–34	10 020
35–39	11 130
40–44	13 125
45–49	15 865
50–54	19 655
55–59	28 120
60–64	46 345
Mean	17 160

*Means for 5 years, 1968–1972. From *Digest of Statistics Analysing Certificates of Incapacity*, HMSO.

The steady increase in days lost with age might merely be a reminder that those ills to which the flesh is heir become more common as one gets older, and the regional variations might be just a crude reflection of the different types of industry in different parts of the country. It is well known, however, that other factors are also involved.

Most absence from work, and especially that of short duration, is voluntary. The patient, in effect, certifies himself as unfit, although he

Table 1.8. Average number of days lost per employee, by cause and by size of unit (number of employees), at 67 works operated by a Public Corporation, 1954*

Size of unit (Number employed)	Number of units	Accidents	Sickness	Other causes	Total
Above 500	4	1.08	15.01	4.43	20.52
200–499	8	0.72	12.83	4.04	17.59
100–199	16	0.88	10.03	2.85	13.75
50–99	12	1.23	11.59	2.57	15.38
25–49	10	0.80	9.76	1.68	12.25
Below 25	17	—	10.88	0.38	11.26

*From R.W. Revans, in *Modern Trends in Occupational Health*, ed. R.S.F. Schilling, 1960.

may require the doctor to act as his agent by signing the appropriate document. Doctors generally are so little acquainted with the demands which their patients' occupations make upon them that they are seldom in the position to evaluate fully a man's fitness to return to work. The liaison between general practitioner and factory doctor is seldom well enough established for the general practitioner to be able to take his colleague's advice and so he relies on the patient to tell him whether or not he is fit to work.

Absence from work is frequently the means by which a man escapes from stress. For example, new employees tend to have more time off work than those with long service and this has been explained by suggesting that the new employee withdraws from work to help him adjust to his new environment. Poor relations between men and management are another cause for high absenteeism. Smaller factories generally have a higher degree of social cohesiveness and as the number of employees increases, so communications become more tortuous, less effective and absenteeism increases (Table 1.8). Monotonous, repetitive work is well recognized to lead to declining morale and a high rate of absenteeism. To some extent the boredom associated with this kind of work can be relieved by putting men onto shift work and in some studies this has been shown to result in a decrease in the amount of lost time (Table 1.9).

Clearly many of the factors which are associated with absenteeism from work can best be resolved by working towards the elimination of stressful conditions, improving communications and relieving boredom. These are all problems which can be tackled by enlightened management in conjunction with industrial psychologists since these problems

Table 1.9. Mean annual rates of absence in matched pairs of day and shift workers for 1968 and 1969 from 29 organizations*

	Certified sickness		Short sickness		Other absence	
	Day	Shift	Day	Shift	Day	Shift
Number of men	965	965	812	812	643	643
Spells/man year	0.77	0.67	1.7	1.41	0.68	0.53
Days/man year	12.13	9.54	2.53	2.11	0.93	0.71
Average length of spell	15.8	14.2	1.5	1.5	1.4	1.3

*From M.L. Newhouse and R.S.F. Schilling, in *Occupational Health Practice*, ed. R.S.F. Schilling, 1973.

are not predominantly medical. Nevertheless, the doctor owes it both to himself and his patient to be aware of the causes for absence from work if only because patients may be more prepared to discuss their problems with their doctor than with management or with colleagues at work.

So far as absence from work for long periods goes, this is usually due to genuine medical or psychiatric conditions and the doctor will help his patient best by having at least some knowledge of the man's occupation and the physical and mental demands which this occupation will impose. Many firms are willing to re-introduce men back into some form of selective employment until they are fit enough to resume their old job. Some of the more forward thinking companies have special rehabilitation units through which men can pass to their old job or in which chronically sick or injured men can work. Doctors outside industry are not likely to become familiar with such arrangements unless they can establish a link with local industrial medical officers or with government agencies such as the Employment Medical Advisory Service (EMAS) in the United Kingdom; it would certainly be in their patients' interest for them to do so, however.

CHAPTER 2/INDUSTRIAL TOXICOLOGY 1: METALS

Although many of the classic occupational diseases caused by exposure to toxic substances are seen much less frequently now in the fully developed industrialized countries, industrial toxicology is nevertheless one of the key stones for an understanding of occupational medicine. In those countries which are rapidly industrializing, occupational diseases are common and occupational medicine could scarcely be practiced in the absence of a sound grounding in toxicology.

The number of potentially toxic materials in use in industry is enormous and so it is possible here to mention only those which are most important and most commonly encountered. In the present chapter, the metals and metalloids (arsenic and phosphorus) are considered; solvents and other organic compounds in Chapters 3 and 4 and the toxic gases in Chapter 5.

Some general considerations of metal toxicology

Within the body, the levels of essential metals are kept within what are referred to as concentration windows. This is because for all these metals there is a concentration below which the signs of deficiency occur and one above which the metal is toxic. The width of the concentration window is thus set by these two extreme levels and in some cases is extremely narrow. In most cases, the metal levels in the body are regulated by uptake from the gut and special absorptive mechanisms have been evolved for this purpose. The general pattern is that metals in the gut bind to a carrier protein in order to cross the gut mucosa; once across they are split from the carrier protein to become attached to a transport (or storage) protein from which ions are released as required. The activation of the transport mechanism is governed by the metal levels in the body, being stimulated by decreasing and inhibited by increasing levels. There are no specific transport mechanisms for non-essential metals, instead they take advantage of those by which the essential metals are absorbed and their rate of uptake is frequently determined by the concentration of other metals in the gut; some specific examples are given below.

All metals within biological systems are in their ionic state although they all exist in combination with ligands to which they are bound more or less firmly depending on their function. For example, Na^+ and K^+ which are both charge carriers, have a residence time with their ligands (water molecules) of about 10^{-10} seconds. Metals which have a predominantly structural function, such as magnesium for example, are very firmly bound and exchange ligands extremely slowly. No metals undergo biotransformation within the body and most are excreted in the urine.

Metals have many functions, but it is possible to recognize some major categories of effect. I have already mentioned that Na^+ and K^+ act as charge carriers and are responsible, *inter alia,* for the propagation of the action potential down the axon. Calcium appears to act as a trigger mechanism for events such as post-synaptic transmission and muscle contraction whilst metals in the first transition series in the period table, which can exist in more than one oxidation state (Fe^{2+}, Fe^{3+}, for example) are involved in redox reactions. Perhaps the most important function of metals, however, is as vital components of metallo-enzymes of which many hundreds are now known. The role of the metal is either to serve as the active site of the enzyme or to maintain the structural integrity of the protein through its binding with amino-acid residues.

An important aspect of metal toxicology is the ability of metals to interact with one another. Interactions between metals may occur because they are adjacent to each other in the periodic table or because their ionic radius or electronic configuration is similar. The interactions may be synergistic or antagonistic and it is the ability of toxic metals to interact with those which are essential which underlies many of their harmful effects. For example cadmium and zinc interact and cadmium is thus able to displace zinc in some metallo-enzymes. Lead can displace calcium at any of the sites at which it is active and thus is able, for example, to inhibit post-synaptic transmission.

Lead

Uses: Lead has many uses in industry including the manufacture of pipes, sheet metal and foil. It is also still used in paints, enamels and glazes, although on a smaller scale than a few years ago. An important use has been connected with the development of the motor industry and great quantities of lead have been used in the manufacture of car batteries, and in making the alkyl lead compounds used as anti-knock additives in petrol. In many countries now the use of lead based antiknock agents is being discontinued because of the supposed behavioural effects of environmental lead on children.

Hazards of use: The predominant hazard in industry arises from the inhalation of dust and fume but the organic compounds may also be absorbed through the skin. Ingestion is a much less serious problem in industry, although in the general environment it is the predominant route of entry.

Metabolism: Inorganic lead is relatively poorly absorbed from the gut, only about 10 per cent of an ingested dose being taken up. The rate of absorption is dependent upon the concentration of other metals in the gut, particularly to those of calcium and iron. Lead uptake varies inversely with the concentration of these metals in the gut, a factor which may be of importance when considering exposure to lead in workers in developing countries. Lead which is present in the faeces is mainly that which has been ingested but not absorbed, although there is a small amount in the faeces which has been excreted through the bile. Pulmonary absorption is much more effective, and, depending on the chemical species and the particle size, about 40 per cent of inhaled lead is absorbed. Organic compounds, including the lead alkyls and lead stearate are absorbed through the skin.

Following absorption, lead is transported bound to the red cell, and considerably less than 10 per cent of the total blood lead concentration represents lead in the plasma. All the soft tissues have their complement of lead, but the skeleton acts as the main depository and more than 90 per cent of the total body burden of lead is in the bones and teeth. Lead displaces calcium in the hydroxyapatite crystal and once within the bone is relatively stable although some exchange does take place between the skeleton and the plasma. Inorganic lead does not normally cross the blood-brain barrier with any ease but organic lead does.

Excretion is almost exclusively via the kidneys but small amounts are lost in addition through the bile and through sweat, and in milk.

Poisoning: The symptoms of lead poisoning include abdominal pain, constipation and vomiting. Peripheral neuropathy is seldom seen in industrial cases nowadays, although in the old text books, wrist drop was always given great prominence. Some patients complain of a metallic taste in the mouth and some complain of headache. There may be clinical signs of anaemia, although this is a late manifestation of the disease. A blue line on the gums due to the deposition of lead sulphide in the gingival margin is occasionally seen. This lead line has come to be regarded as one of the classic signs of lead poisoning but students are warned not to hesitate to make the diagnosis in its absence; they are unlikely to see it! Encephalopathy is an uncommon but serious complication in adults with lead poisoning although conversely, it is often the presenting symptom in children.

Table 2.1. Symptoms in inorganic and organic lead poisoning in adults*

Inorganic	Organic
Abdominal pain	Disturbances in sleep pattern
Constipation	Nausea
Vomiting	Anorexia
Non-abdominal pain	Vomiting
Asthenia	Vertigo and headache
Paraesthesiae	Muscular weakness
Psychological symptoms	Weight loss
Diarrhoea	Tremor
	Diarrhoea
	Abdominal pain
	Hyperexcitability
	Mania

*Symptoms are listed in their order of frequency as presenting symptoms.

Organic lead poisoning may result from exposure to tetraethyl lead (TEL); tetramethyl lead (TML) is much less toxic than TEL and cases of poisoning with TML have not been reported. The symptoms of organic lead poisoning differ from those of inorganic poisoning in that psychiatric manifestations are more common presenting symptoms. For comparison, the symptoms of the two conditions are shown in Table 2.1 in order of their frequency of occurrence.

Inorganic lead poisoning may not be easy to diagnose in the absence of biochemical data. When these are to hand, however, the spectrum of abnormalities is virtually pathognomonic (see below). In the past, patients with inorganic lead poisoning have found themselves in a surgical ward having investigations to establish the cause of their acute abdomen and some have come to laparotomy before the true cause of their illness has been discovered, usually by taking a proper occupational history from the patient. Some care needs to be taken in establishing exposure, however, since in most cases of lead poisoning these days, the patient does not work in a 'traditional' lead industry but may be engaged in demolishing bridges or other buildings covered with lead paint, for example. Anyone who takes a flame to old painted structures should be warned about the possibility of lead exposure and protected accordingly.

The psychiatric symptoms of organic lead poisoning have no characteristics by which their origin may easily be discovered. Patients have been known to develop organic lead poisoning by using leaded petrol as a solvent in confined spaces and cases of encephalopathy have been reported in children and adults sniffing petrol. Some cases of congenital malformation have also been reported in children born to women who sniffed leaded petrol during pregnancy.

Lead anaemia: Anaemia is seen only in inorganic poisoning and occurs late in the disease, but disturbances of haem synthesis can be detected almost as soon as exposure to lead has begun. Lead, like many of the other heavy metals, is a powerful inhibitor of enzymes containing a sulphydryl (—SH) group and a number of these enzymes are concerned with haem synthesis. The disturbances produced by the inhibition of these enzymes form the basis of a number of tests by which the effects of lead on those at risk are monitored (Fig. 2.1). The effects include, reduction in the activity of δ-amino laevulinic acid dehydrase (ALA-d) in the circulating red cells, and increase in the urinary excretion of δ-amino laevulinic acid (ALA) and coproporphyrin (Cp), and an increase in erythrocyte protoporphyrin (EPP). The increase in EPP occurs because lead inhibits the incorporation of Fe^{2+} into the protoporphyrin molecule and its place may be taken by Zn^{2+} with the formation of zinc protoporphyrin (ZPP). The main elevation of EPP levels occurs about 3 months after the change in exposure since it is only the newly formed red cells which are affected. Since the red cell has a life span of about 120 days it follows that it will take that time to replace the normal red cells with those which are rich in protoporphyrin. It is also obvious that it will take about three months for high EPP levels to fall to normal after exposure is discontinued.

There is little or no elevation of the urinary ALA or Cp excretion in organic lead poisoning; nor is the erythrocyte protoporphyrin level much increased; red cell ALA-d activity, however, is significantly decreased.

The inhibition of haem synthesis is one factor in the production of lead anaemia but lead also produces direct effects on the red cell. The permeability of the membrane is altered in such a way as to allow an increased potassium loss from the cell and the life span of the red cell is

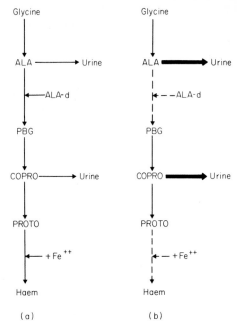

Fig. 2.1. Diagram to show normal haem synthesis (a) and the effects of lead (b).

A number of enzymes are inhibited, the most important of which is ALA-d. As a result the levels of ALA and COPRO in the urine are increased and the activity of ALA-d in the circulating red cells is decreased. The incorporation of Fe^{++} into PROTO is also inhibited. If exposure is continued for a long time, frank anaemia will be produced.

Abbreviations: ALA = δ-amino laevulinic acid; PBG = porphobilinogen; COPRO = coproporphyrin; PROTO = protoporphyrin; ALA-d = δ-amino laevulinic acid dehydrase.

slightly shortened. There are also alterations in iron metabolism and iron-laden cells (siderocytes) may be found in the peripheral blood and in the bone marrow, and the serum iron may be elevated.

In the older books, great store was given to the presence of basophilic stippled cells in the peripheral blood as an index of lead absorption and lead intoxication. The presence of these cells, however, is not specific for lead poisoning. For example, they are also found after exposure to aniline, benzene and carbon monoxide, and as a test for lead absorption, stippled cell counts have been superseded by more sensitive biochemical tests.

Biochemical indices of lead poisoning: The biochemical features of lead poisoning are so characteristic that, when all are present, a diagnosis may be made with confidence. A raised blood lead concentration is essential for the diagnosis and the urinary lead level will also be raised. There will be a marked elevation or urinary ALA and Cp excretion but only a minimal rise in urinary PBG. The erythrocyte protoporphyrin concentration will be raised and the activity of ALA-d greatly inhibited. There is no other disease in which the combination of effects occurs.

Control and treatment: Medical supervision of certain groups of lead workers is mandatory. Women (because of the high incidence of spontaneous abortion and stillbirth in the past) and young persons are prohibited from working in certain processes connected with lead manufacture.

Biological monitoring of lead workers is based on a test of absorption (the blood lead concentration) and a test which measures metabolic effect, either the urinary ALA concentration or the red cell proto-porphyrin concentration. In the control of lead workers, the blood lead concentration is generally given most weight and it is most unlikely that lead poisoning will occur if the level is kept below 80 μg/dl (3.9 μmol/l). Cases of lead poisoning may undoubtedly occur in sensitive individuals when the blood lead is lower than 80 μg/dl but such sensitivity should have been apparent by an unusually great excretion of ALA in the urine or in a markedly elevated EPP. In recent years there has been a tendency to lower the blood lead concentration at which men should be removed from exposure; in the UK and the other countries of the EEC, the suspension limit is now 70 μg/dl. The frequency with which blood lead estimations will be carried out depends on the concentration found. The UK Code of Practice suggests that when the blood lead is less than 40 μg/dl, the maximum interval between tests shall be 12 months, between 40–59 μg/dl the maximum interval shall be 6 months, between 60–69 μg/dl, 3 months and over 70 μg/dl, the interval shall be at the discretion of the supervising physician but not more than 3 months. It should be remembered that the commonest cause of an unusually high blood lead concentration in a worker who has been well-controlled is contamination and before any action is taken, a high reading must be confirmed on another sample.

All operations which give rise to dust or fume should be exhaust ventilated and workers should wear appropriate protective clothing. Where one man in a group, all of whom have approximately the same degree of exposure, shows signs of increased absorption, this may be evidence that local ventilation has failed or that the man is not complying with safety requirements. Both possibilities ought to be investigated.

The combination of laboratory tests, regular clinical examination and good industrial hygiene should be sufficient to protect workers from developing any significant degree of clinical lead poisoning and severe industrial cases are nowadays a rarity in this country. On a world-wide basis, however, lead poisoning is still the most prevalent industrial disease.

Organic poisoning: The total blood lead concentration is not raised in organic lead poisoning, although the fraction which is lipid-bound is usually elevated. It is technically rather difficult to estimate the lipid-bound fraction, and so biological monitoring of organic lead workers tends to be based on urinary lead analyses; the aim should be to keep the urinary lead concentration below 150 $\mu g/l$ (0.7 $\mu mol/l$).

Treatment: Treatment of lead poisoning must be undertaken only in hospital under supervised conditions. Patients with lead colic will gain relief from an intravenous injection of calcium gluconate and other symptoms will be relieved as the blood lead concentration falls. This will happen following removal from exposure but when the fall is slow or when symptoms are slow to resolve then treatment with a chelating agent (calcium-EDTA or pencillamine are most commonly used) may be required.

Mercury

Uses: Metallic mercury is used in the manufacture of thermometers and switch-gear, in the manufacture of amalgams with copper, tin, silver or gold, and of solders containing mercury, tin and lead. It is also used in the chemical industry to produce many mercury compounds, but probably its greatest use is in mercury cell rooms for the manufacture of chlorine.

Inorganic mercury compounds which have an industrial use include the nitrate, used in the 'carrotting' of rabbit fur to form felt for hats, the sulphide, which is used as a red pigment (vermilion) and the red oxide used in the manufacture of the anti-fouling paints which are applied to the bottom of ships.

Of the organic compounds, the ethyl, methyl, phenyl and tolyl compounds are used as seed dressings to prevent the spread of fungicidal seed diseases. They are also used as antislime agents in paper making. Mercury fulminate is used in the manufacture of explosives.

Hazards of use: Risks from metallic mercury occur during mining and recovery of the metal from the ore and during the manufacture of compounds from the metal. The risk is from the inhalation of mercury vapour. Since mercury evaporates at room temperature it maybe a hazard in laboratories if scientific instruments are broken, thus allowing the metal to escape. Substantial quantities of mercury vapour may also be detected in dentists' surgeries. Although both the inhalation and the ingestion of compounds of mercury may occur in industry, inhalation is the major hazard by far. When handling mercury it should be remembered that it may be absorbed through the unbroken skin. Indeed, mercury used to be administered therapeutically by rubbing mercury ointment on the skin.

Of the organic compounds, only the methyl and ethyl derivatives have been reported to produce systemic toxic effects in man. The fulminate is a primary skin irritant but does not readily produce systemic poisoning.

Metabolism: Approximately 80 per cent of inhaled mercury vapour will be absorbed from the lungs. The rate of absorption of inhaled mercury compounds will depend upon their particle size and their chemical composition. Absorption of metallic mercury from the gastro-intestinal tract is negligible, but by contrast, absorption of methyl mercury is virtually complete. Mercurous mercury salts are virtually insoluble and must be oxidized to the mercuric form before absorption is possible. Less than 15 per cent of ingested inorganic mercury salts are absorbed from the gut; the residue being eliminated in the faeces.

After absorption, elemental mercury is widely distributed through the body and is rapidly oxidized to Hg^{2+} in the tissues. The newly oxidized mercury binds to protein and is distributed as inorganic mercury. Elemental mercury is able to cross the blood-brain barrier easily and it also crosses the placenta. Inorganic compounds do not cross the blood-brain barrier but are widely distributed to the other tissues.

Some organic mercury compounds, particularly the phenyl and alkoxyalkyl derivatives are rapidly converted in the liver to the inorganic form. The conversion of ethyl mercury to the inorganic form is slow and the conversion of methyl mercury is virtually non-existent. The organic mercury compounds rapidly penetrate the blood-brain barrier and easily cross the placenta.

The kidney contains by far the greatest concentration of mercury, mainly in the cortical and sub-cortical regions, and 50 per cent or more of the total body burden may be in the kidney. The liver also contains a high concentration of mercury, as will the brain following exposure to elemental mercury or the alkylmercury compounds.

Mercury is excreted in the urine following exposure to elemental mercury, inorganic compounds and aryl or alkoxyalkyl mercury. The principal route for the elimination of methyl mercury is via the faeces, but the excretion rate is slow; the half-life of the alkylmercury compounds in man is estimated to be 70–80 days.

Mercury is also excreted in sweat and in saliva whilst mercury vapour is also eliminated through the lungs.

Methyl mercury passes into breast milk and infants suckling mothers who are heavily exposed may accumulate dangerously high doses; the half-life of alkylmercury compounds in man is estimated to be 70–80 days and that of inorganic mercury to be about 60 days.

Acute poisoning: In industry acute poisoning has usually occurred when workers have been exposed to mercury which has been heated in a confined space. It is a rare condition. The patient presents with an acute febrile illness, the symptoms of which come on some hours after exposure has terminated. Prominent symptoms include cough, dyspnoea, tachypnoea, fever, nausea, vomiting, lethargy and a feeling of tightness in the chest. Some patients develop rigors and some are cyanosed. In mild cases the symptoms resolve spontaneously, although dyspnoea and tightness in the chest may persist for up to a week, and sometimes longer. Severe cases may require admission to hospital and treatment on a respirator.

Fatal cases show a pathological picture of acute diffuse interstitial fibrosis with a profuse fibrinous exudate and erosion of the lining of the bronchi and bronchioles.

Acute poisoning may also occur from the accidental ingestion of a large quantity of a mercury compound, and in the past, cases were reported following the application of mercury for therapeutic purposes. Following ingestion, the symptoms include gastric pain, nausea and vomiting, shock, and in fatal cases, syncope with convulsions, leading to coma.

Chronic poisoning: The most serious effects of chronic mercury poisoning are produced on the nervous system, on behaviour and on the kidney. Symptoms of chronic mercurialism may be caused by both inorganic and organic compounds, but psychiatric symptoms tend to predominate over neurological in inorganic poisoning whereas the converse is true in organic poisoning. The earliest symptoms are vague, and include the development of a sallow complexion, dyspepsia and headaches. Gingivitis and excessive salivation are early symptoms. The teeth may become loose and drop out, leaving those which remain blackened and eroded. A 'mercury line' may be seen rarely on the gums. This resembles the blue 'lead line', but is more often dark brown in colour. Chronic exposure to organic mercury compounds produces skin lesions. The fulminate is particularly notorious in this respect, giving rise to an irritant dermatitis (fulminate itch) and discrete ulcers (powder holes).

Neurological signs: The characteristic disturbance in chronic mercury poisoning is the production of a tremor, which is neither as fine nor as regular as that found in thyrotoxicosis. It begins as an intention tremor in the hands but later affects the eyelids, lips and tongue, finally involving the arms and sometimes also the legs. As it progresses the tremor becomes coarsened and its amplitude is exaggerated if attention is drawn to it. The tremor is known colloquially as the hatters' shakes. Accompanying the tremor there is often a characteristic disturbance of the handwriting which becomes progressively tremulous, irregular and unintelligible. Various speech disorders are found in addition. These include, hesitancy in beginning sentences and a difficulty in pronunciation and both are more severe in organic than in inorganic poisoning.

Motor and sensory nerve disorders are also part of the neurological syndrome. Spastic gait is a feature and cerebellar ataxia may be severe especially in organic poisoning. Hyperactive tendon reflexes, especially the knee jerk, may be elicited and the plantar reflexes may be extensor.

Sensory disturbances include paraesthesiae, alteration in taste and smell, and loss of proprioception in the fingers and the toes. Touch and pain modalities, on the other hand, may be normal. Some patients have difficulty in hearing unless the words are spoken slowly and deliberately and actual hearing loss has been found many years after an acute episode of poisoning. In organic poisoning there is a gross peripheral constriction of the visual fields.

The most important pathological lesion found in fatal cases is atrophy of the cerebellar cortex, which accounts for many of the signs and symptoms found during life.

There is some evidence that sub-clinical neuropsychiatric symptoms can be detected in mercury workers; defects in recent memory have been found in those whose urinary mercury levels have been elevated (> 50 μg/g creatinine) for several months, for example. In one study, speed of foot tapping was found to be inversely related to urinary mercury concentration and when the urinary mercury levels were lowered by removing the workers from exposure, the foot tapping speed returned to normal. Finally, some reports indicate that sensory nerve conduction velocities are low in mercury workers even in the absence of any overt clinical signs.

Erethism: This is a form of toxic organic psychosis which was once common in the hat industry, hence the expression, 'mad as a hatter'. It is described as an abnormal state of timidity and can present as an anxiety neurosis. Later, however, features of an organic syndrome, including irritability, apathy, drowsiness and headaches frequently develop. Less frequently, dementia and psychotic symptoms may point to the organic nature of the syndrome. When first noted, the emotional disorder may be accompanied by signs of vaso-motor disturbance, including blushing, excessive perspiration and dermatographia.

Effects on the kidney: Proteinuria may be found in up to 5 per cent of men chronically exposed to mercury but usually disappears when exposure is discontinued. In a few cases however, it persists and progresses towards chronic renal disease.

The nephrotic syndrome has been reported in workers exposed to mercury and is said to remit completely when exposure is discontinued. It is not certain that this is always the case, however.

Mercurialentis: Examination of the lens with a slit lamp may reveal a brownish coloured reflex from the anterior capsule. This brown colour becomes deeper as exposure is prolonged. It is usually accompanied by fine punctate opacities in the lens but neither these nor the discoloration has any effect on visual acuity. The chief value of this sign is as an indication of prolonged exposure to mercury for forensic purposes, although the sign may appear within a few months of exposure.

Environmental mercury poisoning: There have been a number of large-scale outbreaks of environmental methyl mercury poisoning. The most notorious was the Minamata Bay episode in Japan. A factory manu-facturing vinyl chloride using mercuric chloride as a catalyst discharged its effluent into the bay where some of the mercury was methylated by aquatic micro-organisms; the methyl mercury produced entered the food chain and the residents were poisoned through eating con-taminated fish. In Iraq, mass poisonings have resulted from the eating of seed grains treated with methyl and ethyl mercury. Grain is treated in this way before planting to guard against disease; it ought never to be eaten, as these tragic episodes amply demonstrated.

Treatment: Treatment of mercury poisoning with chelating agents, BAL and Ca-EDTA has been tried with varying success. Some improvement in symptomatology can be expected after exposure has ceased but poisoning from inorganic mercury may take many weeks to resolve. Patients suffering from organic poisoning will require intensive physiotherapy and speech therapy, but even so, some permanent disabilities are almost certain.

Cadmium

Uses: Cadmium is a constituent of some alloys used to manufacture bearings for motor car and other engines and the manufacture of these alloys accounts for most of the cadmium used in industry. It is also used as a protective coating for iron, steel and copper in the electroplating industry and it is replacing zinc to some extent as a rust-proofing agent for iron and steel. The negative plates of alkaline storage batteries are made from cadmium and it is incorporated in cadmium vapour lamps. In nuclear reactors it is used as a neutron absorber, either as a coating on graphite or in the form of rods. Cadmium sulphide is used to prepare yellow and orange pigments and cadmium selenosulphide is used to make red pigments. The pigments, in turn, are used for colouring inks, paints and a variety of plastic, rubber, glass and enamel ware.

Hazards of use: The principal industrial hazards arise from the smelting of ores, the welding and melting of cadmium plated metals, the manufacture of alkaline batteries and the preparation of pigments. In all these cases the risk is from inhalation of cadmium (or cadmium oxide) vapour or dust. Ingestion is seldom a hazard in industry.

Metabolism: The absorption of cadmium from the gut is poor, only about 5–10 per cent of an ingested dose being taken up. The rate of uptake may be enhanced, however, in individuals with low iron stores (as measured by serum ferritin levels). The rate of absorption from the lungs is greater than from the gut and up to 40 per cent of an inhaled dose may be taken up. Significant amounts of cadmium may enter the lungs from the inhalation of tobacco smoke and thus smoking will add to the total exposure in cadmium workers.

Following absorption, cadmium induces the formation of metallothionein, a low molecular weight protein. Metallothionein has a very high proportion of sulphur-containing amino-acids in its structure and its physiological function is to regulate tissue levels of essential metals,

especially zinc and copper. Cadmium is incorporated into metallothionein because its metabolism is similar to that of zinc and about
80–90 per cent of cadmium in the body is bound to metallothionein.
The cadmium-metallothionein complex is transported to the kidney
and filtered through the glomerulus to be resorbed by the cells of the
proximal tubule. In these cells, the protein is broken down by proteases
with the release of free cadmium ions. The presence of these free ions
induces the cells of the proximal tubule to produce more metallothionein which binds the cadmium ions once more. It is generally
considered that kidney damage occurs when the capacity of the tubular
cells to produce metallothionein is surpassed, although, when injected
into animals, the cadmium-metallothionein complex itself is
nephrotoxic.

The half-life of cadmium in the body is long, of the order of 7–30
years and its excretion is slow. The main route of excretion is through
the kidneys but only when the kidney is damaged and its function
impaired does cadmium enter the urine in any quantity. Cadmium
accumulates preferentially in the kidney and liver and only to a limited
degree in the other soft tissues.

Acute poisoning: Following ingestion, symptoms appear suddenly, normally within 2 hours. Symptoms include increased salivation, severe
nausea and persistent vomiting sometimes with haematemesis. Shock
and collapse may follow and diarrhoea and tenesmus supervene at a later
stage. Recovery is also rapid and is usually complete within 24 hours. No
treatment is required beyond the replacement of lost fluids.

Following inhalation of cadmium fumes the symptoms are those of
acute pulmonary irritation accompanied by dyspnoea. During the time
of exposure the patient experiences symptoms which are reminiscent of
those of metal fume fever (*q.v.*). There is some irritation in the throat
and a cough but otherwise no ill effects are noted. This 'latent period'
may last for up to 10 hours when an influenza-like illness suddenly sets
in. In this stage there is severe dyspnoea, cough (which may be uncontrollable), anorexia, nausea, weakness, headaches, diarrhoea, epigastric
pain and malaise. There may be a rise in temperature, and proteinuria
may be detected. This acute stage lasts anything from 1 day to several
weeks and during all this time basal crepitations can be heard in both
lungs and there is radiological evidence of bilateral pulmonary infiltration.

Recovery is gradual and complete in most cases. Fatalities may occur
as the result of severe pulmonary oedema with central cyanosis, and at

post-mortem, proliferative lesions are noted in the alveoli, sometimes completely obliterating the alveolar spaces. An alternative form of death may be due to renal cortical necrosis.

Chronic poisoning: Men with chronic cadmium poisoning may complain of non-specific symptoms such as fatigue, weight loss, gastro-intestinal pain, nausea and persistent cough. Signs of chronic cadmium poisoning include yellow rings on the teeth, anosmia, and a mild hypochromic anaemia due to interference with normal iron and copper metabolism. The major effects of chronic cadmium poisoning, however, are directed against the kidneys and the lungs.

Renal effects: The nephrotoxic effect is directed mainly against the tubules and occurs when the renal cadmium concentration is greater than 200 mg/kg weight. Renal damage is manifested by the excretion of low molecular weight proteins in the urine of which the major constituents are β_2 microglobulins, sometimes used as a means of biological monitoring. Glycosuria and aminoaciduria also occur and there may be a reduced ability to concentrate the urine or to excrete an acid load. Stone formation has been found together with a high rate of phosphate clearance and hypercalcuria.

In spite of these changes, renal failure is practically unknown but the alteration in calcium metabolism consequent upon the hypercalcuria may, in rare cases, lead to osteomalacia.

Effects on the lungs: Chronic exposure to cadmium results in the development of focal emphysema. Bullae are not formed and bronchitis is not a feature. The effects on the lungs are evident long before renal damage is observed and are manifested by the onset of dyspnoea and by a low gas transfer factor. Cadmium has been shown experimentally to reduce the concentration of α_1-antitrypsin in the plasma and this effect may underlie the production of emphysema in cadmium workers.

Prostatic carcinoma: Cadmium workers were at one time considered to have an enhanced risk of prostatic carcinoma but recent epidemiological surveys have failed to confirm this. The prevailing view now is that neither prostatic carcinoma nor any other malignant disease are unusually prevalent amongst men exposed to cadmium at work.

Hypertension: Cadmium can induce hypertension in experimental animals and there is some evidence that the absorption of cadmium from the general environent may be aetiologically related to hypertension in man. This evidence is by no means unequivocal and hypertension is not a risk amongst cadmium workers, nor does it occur in itai-itai disease.

Itai-itai disease: This disease is a painful type of osteomalacia in which multiple fractures and renal dysfunction were features. It occurred amongst elderly multiparous women in Japan and has generally been considered to be due to eating rice contaminated with cadmium from irrigation water which passed through old mining areas. The pathogenesis of the disease is now in some doubt because it has been found in areas where environmental pollution with cadmium does not take place and it has been suggested that it may be a form of vitamin D deficiency.

Treatment: Chelation therapy with CaEDTA has been successfully tried in some patients with acute poisoning. In chronic poisoning the pulmonary and renal changes are unlikely to be noticed until there is severe, irreversible damage.

Beryllium

Uses: Beryllium is used as an alloy with copper. The addition of 2–3 per cent of the metal to copper produces an alloy which is hard, corrosion-resistant, nonrusting and nonsparking. This alloy has a much greater tensile strength than copper alone but its electrical conductivity is approximately the same. Alloys with aluminium, magnesium and nickel are also of commercial value.

Beryllium was formerly used as a constituent of the phosphorescent powder used in fluorescent lights and neon lights. The toxic effects of the metal caused its use in fluorescent lights to be abandoned, but elsewhere its use is increasing. The metal has a high modulus of elasticity and is thus able to resist stress. It imparts lightness, hardness and heat resistance to other materials and is becoming widely used in space research, for example, in the building of space capsules. In nuclear research it is also a valuable material since it gives off α-particles when bombarded with neutrons and it is widely used for cans and other accessories in nuclear reactors. It is also used as a deoxidizer in steel making and as a refractory in crucible making. Pure beryllium foil is used in the windows of X-ray diffraction tubes.

Hazards of use: A hazard from fume and dust occurs during the processes of crushing and extracting the ore and when the briquettes containing the extracted metal in the form of a copper alloy are crushed and heated. A considerable hazard used to exist in the handling of the powdered beryllium compounds used for making the phosphor for fluorescent lights and in the salvaging of these lamps.

Metabolism: Absorption from the gut is poor and 96 per cent or more of ingested beryllium is eliminated in the faeces. Pulmonary absorption, on the other hand, is efficient and rapid. Once absorbed, the beryllium is protein bound and deposited in the liver, spleen and the skeleton and a small residue remains in the lungs. The rate of urinary excretion depends on how rapidly and in what form the beryllium was absorbed.

Acute poisoning: The symptoms of acute poisoning are those of a chemical pneumonitis. There is a cough with blood-stained sputum, retrosternal pain, anorexia, rapidly-increasing fatigue and progressive dyspnoea accompanied by cyanosis. The histological appearances in the lung are those of a lobular pneumonia with the alveoli filled with exudate containing large numbers of plasma cells but few polymorphs. Radiographic changes are minimal in the early stages of the disease but in persistent cases increased linear markings and a diffuse ground-glass appearance may be noted. In addition to the pulmonary manifestations, the patient may have conjunctivitis, rhinitis and pharyngitis. Complete recovery within 1–3 months after removal from exposure is the rule, but fatalities have occurred.

Skin manifestations: Beryllium salts may affect the skin in a number of different ways. They may cause primary irritation, producing a lesion with the appearance of a mild acid burn or they may produce allergic contact dermatitis. The latter is caused mainly by beryllium fluoride and manifests itself by the sudden appearance of intense pruritus and erythema, often accompanied by periorbital oedema. Chemical ulcers develop if beryllium fluoride is allowed to come into contact with broken skin whilst the implantation of beryllium salts under the skin will result in the formation of a subcutaneous granuloma. The implantation of pure beryllium under the skin does not cause granulomata to form.

Not all beryllium compounds affect the skin to an equal degree; beryllium fluoride and sulphate are the most reactive whereas beryllium metal, and the pure oxide and hydroxide are harmless to the skin.

Chronic poisoning: Chronic beryllium poisoning produces a sarcoid-like reaction with the formation of granulomatous lesions in the lungs and other organs. The condition does not occur in those who handle only the pure metal or those whose only exposure is to the ores beryl and bertrandite. There is a latent period ranging from a few weeks to several years between first exposure and the onset of symptoms which develop in an insidious manner. The first sign of anything untoward is a dry, nonproductive cough, accompanied by loss of weight and fatigue. The loss of weight may be dramatic and is often the reason for the patient seeking medical advice. Progressive dyspnoea is the most serious and most distressing symptom of the disease. Tachycardia may be noted on physical examination and the fingers may be clubbed.

The radiological appearances include a fine diffuse granularity with hilar lymph node enlargement. Nodules, varying in size from 1–5 mm are noted and may give a 'snow storm' appearance. The nodules may coalesce to form large opacities, especially in the upper lobes. At a late stage in the disease basal emphysema is noted and this may lead to the development of a small pneumothorax. The signs of cor pulmonale are to be expected as the disease progresses.

Table 2.2. Classification of histological changes found in chronic beryllium poisoning

	Interstitial cellular infiltration	Granulomata	Areas of focal calcification
Group I			
A B	Moderate to marked	Poorly formed or absent / Well formed	Frequently present and numerous
Group II	Slight or absent	Numerous and well formed	Few or absent

From D.G. Freiman and H.L. Hardy, *Human Pathology*, 1, 25, 1970.

Histologically, chronic granulomata are found in the lungs resembling those found in sarcoidosis and similar lesions are also found in the skin, in lymph nodes and in the liver. The granulomata may be well or poorly formed and giant cells are found, as in sarcoid. The predominant cell type is the histiocyte, with lesser numbers of plasma cells and lymphocytes also present. There may be areas of focal calcification, the so-called Schaumann bodies. On the basis of the histological appearance, the lesions can be classified into three groups (Table 2.2). The prognosis seems to be best for patients falling into Group II than for those in either of the sub-groups of Group I.

Neighbourhood poisoning: Cases of beryllium poisoning in individuals living in the vicinity of a beryllium-using factory have been reported. This situation is analogous to that which has arisen in connection with asbestos and poses grave problems both to industrial users and to those concerned with environmental health.

Diagnosis and treatment: The diagnosis of beryllium poisoning depends upon a history of exposure to the metal and the demonstration of beryllium in the urine or in some tissue, either the skin or the lung. The presence of beryllium in the urine indicates that exposure has taken place, but because the rate of excretion is variable, does not indicate the degree of exposure. Most patients with the disease have a positive lymphocyte transformation test to beryllium, and a positive macrophage inhibition test.

Berylliosis may be differentiated from sarcoidosis by the fact that the latter condition may be accompanied by uveitis, involvement of the salivary and lacrimal glands, erythema nodosum, lupus pernio, cystic changes in the bones and by a positive Kveim test. None of these is seen in berylliosis. Moreover, the radiological changes in sarcoid may resolve spontaneously; this is never the case in beryllium poisoning.

Chelation therapy with EDTA has been successfully tried in some patients with acute poisoning. In chronic poisoning the pulmonary changes are unlikely to be noted until there is severe, irreversible damage, but the disease process can be halted with corticosteroids. The prognosis in chronic beryllium poisoning has improved in recent years. Nowadays deaths from the disease are rare, whereas at one time it carried a mortality rate of about 33 per cent. Patients are often left with permanent respiratory impairment, however, but most will be able to work although they are often forced to take a light job. Men with established disease should not, of course, be further exposed.

Manganese

Uses: Manganese is used principally in the manufacture of steel alloys, since its addition to steel greatly enhances its hardness and tensile strength. Ferromanganese is added during the process of steel making to prevent the formation of iron oxide and iron sulphide in the finished product. Other alloys are made with copper, zinc and aluminium. Manganese also has a use in the manufacture of dry cell batteries, whilst in the glass and ceramics industries it is used to remove the green and yellow colours due to traces of iron. Manganese pigments are used in the manufacture of paints, varnishes and dyes, especially those used in calico printing, and it is used in glass-making to colour glass violet. Methylcyclopentadienyl manganese tricarbonyl (MMT) is used as a smoke inhibitor in fuel oil and as an antiknock agent in petrol to supplement lead alkyls.

Hazards of use: The commonest source of hazard arises during the mining and crushing of the ores and the handling of the resultant manganese oxide. Reduction of the dioxide to produce the metal carries a risk of exposure to fume. In the manufacture of batteries and paints the dioxide is handled as a dry dust which presents a hazard in the absence of adequate safety measures.

Metabolism: Manganese is an essential trace mineral. The rate of absorption of inorganic manganese from the gut is very slow and in the trace amounts in which it is present in food, the manganese is probably in the form of organic chelates which are absorbed more avidly. The occupational hazard is thus due to inhaled manganese, although manganese tricarbonyls are absorbed through the skin. Following absorption, plasma clearance is rapid and the metal tends to accumulate in tissues rich in mitochondria, mainly the liver, but also in the kidney; a small amount is present in bone.

The main homeostatic mechanism for regulating the levels of manganese in the body is by biliary excretion and thus elimination is almost exclusively through the faeces. Less than 1 per cent of the daily intake appears in the urine and even after a large intravenous dose, little is excreted through the kidney. MMT, by contrast, is excreted through the urine to a considerable degree.

Acute poisoning: Manganese dioxide fume is irritant to the mucosa of the respiratory tract and may produce pharyngitis or bronchitis. No permanent sequelae are noted although workers exposed to manganese were reported as having an abnormally high risk from pneumonia which does not differ from the usual type except in its slow response to treatment. This view, however, is not generally accepted.

Chronic poisoning: The onset of manganese poisoning is slow and early symptoms are nonspecific. They include headache, lassitude, somnolence and pains in the joints and muscles. Some cases show emotional lability, with a tendency to purposeless weeping or laughing. Others appear hypomanic with flight of ideas, impulsiveness and euphoria but the presence of visual hallucinations point to the organic nature of the syndrome.

Neurological signs are a prominent feature and are due to damage of the basal ganglia, and they closely resemble those of Parkinson's disease. Patients display the typical facies and some have a festinant gait, whilst others have a curious high-stepping gait, the so-called 'hen step'. There is a marked tremor, more prominent in the upper limbs and this may affect the handwriting, but true ataxia is uncommon. The speech is monotonous, with poor articulation and pauses between words, and in severe cases there may be complete aphonia. Sensory changes are not prominent but excessive salivation and perspiration have been noted. Some patients develop a less severe form of the disease which is characterized by an impairment of movement of the muscles of the trunk, making rising from a supine or sitting position difficult. This form of the disease is accompanied by none of the other signs or symptoms described above.

Pathologically there is atrophy of the basal ganglia with internal hydrocephalus. The damage to the basal ganglia embraces the globus pallidus, the lenticular and caudate nuclei, the putamen and the thalamus.

Manganese pneumonia: Men engaged in smelting manganese ores or in making potassium permanganate from manganese oxide are reported to be particularly prone to develop lobar pneumonia. The disease does not differ from that seen in other persons except that it is more resistant to treatment with antibiotics. There are no permanent sequelae and fibrotic changes in the lungs are not noted.

Treatment: Removal from exposure leads to recovery from acute poisoning. Mild cases of chronic poisoning may show some resolution of their psychiatric symptoms after exposure is discontinued. The effectiveness of EDTA in treating chronic poisoning is not encouraging, but most patients with Parkinsonian symptoms are greatly helped by L-dopa.

Chromium

Uses: Chromium is used for the production of alloys with nickel and molybdenum and in making corrosion-resistant steels. It is also used for chromium plating, as a tanning agent in the leather industry and as a pigment in paints and inks, and in rubber and ceramics.

Hazards of use: These arise from any processes which involve the handling of the metal or its compounds. During the process of chromium plating, a chromic-acid mist is produced which is a potential hazard if the local exhaust ventilation on the plating tank is working inefficiently.

Metabolism: Chromium is an essential trace element required for glucose metabolism. Absorption from the gut depends upon the chemical form which is ingested: less than 1 per cent of trivalent chromium is absorbed, whereas for hexavalent compounds, this value rises to 50 per cent. The rate of absorption from the lung is unknown, although considerable quantities are retained there and the lungs are amongst the organs which normally contain the highest concentration of chromium. The metal is rapidly removed from the blood and is excreted predominantly in the urine. At least 80 per cent of chromium is excreted via the kidney, the remainder appears in the faeces.

Poisoning: The trivalent chromium, which binds to organic molecules, is toxic although ironically, workers exposed to hexavalent compounds are most at risk because the hexavalent compounds are much more readily absorbed.

The skin is the organ chiefly affected by chrome and the lesions produced are described in Chapter 7. The nasal mucosa may become ulcerated and this is a hazard which is experienced principally by those engaged in chrome-plating operations. As a rule the ulceration is painless and is discovered during a medical examination. The cartilaginous part of the septum only is affected and it may become perforated. Malignant change does not supervene.

Inflammation of the larynx with ulceration has been described and a pneumonitis can occur with exposure to high concentrations of chromic acid mist. In a few cases, asthmatic symptoms have been described in men exposed to chrome.

Carcinoma of the lung has an increased incidence amongst chromate workers and this association is referred to again in the chapter on occupational cancer.

Zinc

Uses: Zinc is used as a rust-proof coating for iron and steel, in the manufacture of alloys and, in the form of sheet, as a case for batteries, etc. The oxide and the sulphide are used in the dyestuffs and paint industries, and the chloride is used in soldering fluxes. Brass contains copper and from 5–40 per cent of zinc.

Hazards of use: The chief hazard is from the inhalation of zinc oxide fume which is generated when the metal is heated above its melting point. Zinc chloride fumes in heavy concentrations can be toxic, even lethal.

Metabolism: Zinc is an essential metal. It is poorly absorbed from the gut and excreted mainly in the faeces. Just as with iron, the kidneys play little part in regulating body stores. There are a number of zinc-containing enzymes of which the first to be identified was carbonic anhydrase. Zinc is vital for the proper functioning of these enzymes but in addition, it also seems to be necessary in the process of wound healing. It has been suggested that the indolent ulcers on Henry VIII's legs were a consequence of his state of zinc deficiency.

Poisoning: Inhalation of zinc oxide fume gives rise to the syndrome known as metal-fume fever. Other metals can produce the syndrome, including copper, magnesium, which with zinc are the commonest causes, but aluminium, antimony, cadmium, iron, silver and copper are also culpable. The symptoms are recognized in a number of industries, hence the many synonyms for the disease, brassfounders' ague, brass chills, smelter shakes, zinc chills, galvanizers' poisoning, copper fever, foundry fever, Monday fever and the smothers.

The symptoms, which resemble those of influenza, include chills, fever, headaches, nausea, thirst, cough and pain in the limbs. There is usually a leucocytosis of $12.0–16.0 \times 10^9/l$. Recovery is rapid, usually within 24 hours and always within 48 hours. There are no sequelae. Men who work continuously with zinc develop an immunity to attacks which is quickly lost. It is for this reason that the attacks are more prevalent on Mondays after a week-end away from work.

Zinc chloride fumes are toxic in high concentrations, producing dyspnoea, retrosternal and epigastric pain, stridor and cough with expectoration. Fatalities have been recorded.

Zinc stearate: Fatalities following the inhalation of zinc stearate have occurred in infants, and occupational exposure may cause redness and irritation of the mucous membranes of the nose, but the material is generally not regarded as being unduly toxic.

Nickel

Uses: Nickel is used in the production of a number of alloys, including special steels. So-called silver coins are, in fact, made from an alloy of copper and nickel, whilst with zinc and copper, nickel forms the basis of silver-plated tableware, etc.—EPNS. Finely divided nickel is used as a catalyst, especially in the hydrogenation of oils to solid fats. The metal is also used to make enamels and is a constituent of nickel-cadmium batteries. Nickel salts (of which nickel sulphate is the most important) are widely used in electroplating, and all chrome plated products have an under-layer of nickel which is several times the thickness of the chrome finish.

Metabolism: Nickel is poorly absorbed from the gut, but once absorbed, is widely distributed. The lungs and the brain show the highest concentrations. Excretion is rapid through both the urine and the faeces.

Hazards of use: All those who handle nickel or its salts are liable to be at risk.

Poisoning: Nickel and its salts are notorious for producing contact dermatitis, particularly in women who are exposed to nickel in jewellery and in fasteners for various items of clothing. Outside industry, nickel dermatitis is very rarely seen in men. A greater hazard to life is the production of carcinoma of the nasal passages and air sinuses which have been related to nickel exposure. The most toxic nickel-containing substance is nickel carbonyl which will be discussed with the gases in Chapter 5.

Vanadium

Uses: Much of the vanadium used in industry goes to the manufacture of special steel alloys, because the addition of small amounts of vanadium greatly increases the tensile strength of steel. It is also a major element in high-strength titanium alloys. Vanadium salts are used also as catalysts in chemical processes, the most important being vanadium pentoxide, in the production of sulphuric acid. Vanadium compounds are also used in the manufacture of dyes, inks, paints and varnishes.

Hazards of use: Hazards may arise during the crushing of the ores when dust may be inhaled. Most cases of poisoning, however, have occurred during the cleaning of oil-fired burners or gas turbines. Vanadium occurs in all fuel oils but the amount of the metal in the ash depends upon the geographical origin of the crude oil. Venezualan oil contains most and there may be as much as 45 per cent of vanadium in ash from such oil. Vanadium is a constituent of the blood pigment of sea squirts and sea cucumbers which pass their life fixed to rocks and the fossilized remains of these creatures account for the vanadium present in crude oil.

Metabolism: Vanadium is poorly absorbed from the gut and even if soluble salts are ingested, only about 1 per cent of the dose is taken up. Excretion via the kidney is extremely rapid and the metal is not stored to any appreciable degree in the body although it has been noted that concentrations in the lung tend to increase with age.

Poisoning: The toxic effects of vanadium are the result of inflammation of the mucous membranes. Thus conjunctivitis, nasal catarrh and bronchitis are prominent initial symptoms. There may be soreness in the throat and chest and the patient has a dry cough. Wheezing and dyspnoea of effort appear at a later stage, usually within 6–24 hours after first exposure. A tremor of the fingers and hands may be present and some patients complain of depression. The characteristic feature of vanadium intoxication is a greenish-black discoloration of the tongue. The colour disappears within 2–3 days after exposure is discontinued.

Eczematous lesions of the skin have been noted and it is suggested that workers should be batch tested with 2 per cent sodium vanadate before being allowed into contact with the metal.

There are no long-term sequelae of vanadium poisoning although it is said that those who inhale the metal have an increased susceptibility to bronchitis and pneumonia.

Treatment: Fortunately none is required since complete, rapid recovery is the rule.

Phosphorus

Phosphorus presents as an industrial hazard in one of four forms, as yellow phosphorus, as tri-ortho-cresyl phosphate, as organic phosphorus insecticides and as phosphine which is discussed in Chapter 5.

Yellow Phosphorus

Uses: Yellow phosphorus is one of the three allotropes of phosphorus and the only one which is poisonous. Red phosphorus is made from yellow phosphorus and used in the manufacture of matches and fireworks. Yellow phosphorus is generally banned for the manufacture of all but war goods, where its incendiary properties lend themselves to the manufacture of explosives and so on.

Phosphorus compounds are used in the manufacture of detergents, in paper-making, printing and in the manufacture of soaps and dyes. The fertilizer industry uses vast quantities of phosphorus compounds in producing super-phosphate, and metaphosphates are widely used as water softeners.

Hazards of use: Yellow phosphorus bursts into flame at a temperature of $30°C$, burning to form dense white clouds of phosphorus pentoxide. It must never be picked up by the fingers since it will produce painful burns which are slow to heal. In contact with air it oxidizes to form phosphorus trioxide and possibly the pentoxide, the fumes of which are poisonous.

Poisoning: Yellow phosphorus was once widely used to make matches but this practice was banned by the Berne Convention of 1906. Phosphorus sesquisulphide is used as a harmless substitute for 'non-safety' matches. The condition which used to affect those engaged in match dipping was known as 'phossy jaw'.

Phossy jaw was an extensive necrosis, usually of the mandible, which developed after a latent interval of anything up to 5 years after first exposure. The condition was heralded by the onset of toothache in a carious tooth. A dull red spot which could be found on the buccal mucosa at this early stage was pathognomonic of the disease. As the disease progressed, the jaw swelled and became painful. The teeth became loose and sinuses formed from the necrotic cavities in the jaw which often contained large sequestra. The sinuses discharged chronically and the whole jaw was often eventually involved in the disease process. The victim was terribly disfigured and a burden to himself and to others on account of the foul smell of the pus which formed as the necrotic bone became infected. The secondary infection sometimes brought about death by spread to the meninges but septicaemia was the more common terminal event and the overall case mortality rate was about 20 per cent. Excision of the jaw was the only treatment which could be offered to the patient and the operation might entail the removal of the whole mandible. Bones other than the lower jaw were affected and this involvement was frequently brought to light through the development of spontaneous fractures.

Yellow phosphorus continues to be used for making weapons of war and great care is now taken during its handling. Nevertheless, minor cases of phossy jaw still occur, but are detected early and the gross case is more likely to trouble the candidate in a pathology examination than the practising occupational physician.

Organic phosphorus insecticides

These compounds are structurally related to di-iso-propylfluoro phosphate and, like it, are powerful irreversible ChE inhibitors. Since 1945 many new compounds have been elaborated and produced on a large scale. Those which are scheduled under the Agriculture (Poisonous Substances) Act of 1952 are shown in Table 2.3.

Table 2.3. Organo-phosphorus insecticides scheduled under the Agriculture (Poisonous Substances) Act, 1952

Amiton and its salts	Mevinphos
Azinphos-ethyl	Mipafox
Azinphos-methyl	Oxydemeton-methyl
Chlorfenvinphos	Parathion
Demeton	Phenkapton
Demeton-methyl	Phorate
Demeton-s-methyl	Phosphamidon
Dichlorvos	Schradan
Dimefox	Sulfotep
Disulfoten	TEPP
Ethion	Thionazin
Mazidox	Vamidothion
Mecarbam	

Metabolism: Organo-phosphorus compounds are readily absorbed through the skin as well as by inhalation and ingestion. They do not accumulate in the body and most are rapidly degraded and excreted. The degradation products, being water-soluble are excreted in the urine; very little of the unchanged compounds appear in the urine. In some cases, the process of degradation produces metabolites which are more toxic than the parent compound. For example, malaoxon and paroxon are more toxic than malathion and parathion from which they derive respectively.

Poisoning: The toxic properties of these compounds to man relate to their anti-ChE activity and depend upon the speed and degree of the ChE inhibition. Toxic symptoms appear when ChE activity is reduced to less than 50 per cent of normal. When parathion was introduced on a large scale its dangers were not fully appreciated and careless use and sloppy handling resulted in several cases of poisoning.

Early signs of poisoning are not specific and include headache, nausea, anorexia and a marked lassitude. Constriction of the pupils may occur and all the symptoms are aggravated by smoking. In a short time following exposure these relatively mild symptoms are superseded by vomiting, diarrhoea, abdominal pain and muscle twitching. Incontinence of urine and faeces is common. Pulmonary oedema is a frequent finding. The onset of convulsions usually signifies that the patient is about to pass into a coma which may lead to his death. The complete course from exposure to death may take as little as an hour so that speed is of the essence if treatment is to be successful.

Treatment with atropine should be given immediately and the patient supported with mechanical respiration if necessary. Cholinesterase activity can be restored by compounds which split the enzyme from its attachment to the phosphate group of the insecticide. Pralidoxime (P2S of P2AM) is satisfactory for this purpose, and a number of hospitals hold supplies of this drug and maintain a 24 hour service.

Late sequelae of poisoning with organo-phosphorus compounds have been noted. The patient recovers from the acute phase but about 3 weeks later notes progressive muscular weakness and fatigue with vomiting and diarrhoea. Marked muscle wasting may follow. The symptoms are similar to those of TOCP poisoning.

To avoid these late complications, all patients who have an attack of acute poisoning should be kept under observation until their blood cholinesterase activity has returned to normal.

Chronic effects: Neuromuscular function and nerve conduction velocities are altered in some workers with prolonged exposure to organo-phosphorus compounds but the significance of these findings is uncertain. There is also some evidence to suggest that prolonged exposure may impair renal tubular function.

Prevention: Those using organo-phosphorus insecticides scheduled under the 1952 Act are obliged by law to be issued with and to wear protective clothing. No man is allowed to work with them for more than 10 hours in 1 day or 60 hours in 7 days. No one under the age of 18 may work with them at all.

Those at risk should have periodic tests of their blood cholinesterase activity, or alternatively have nerve conduction velocities measured. There is a good correlation between urinary excretion of p-nitrophenol and exposure to parathion and this fact may also be made use of in screening programmes. It is also helpful to conduct periodic clinical or radiological examinations of the chest, since the finding of pulmonary oedema without any evidence of cardiac enlargement in an otherwise fit agricultural worker should raise the possibility of intoxication.

Arsenic

Uses: Arsenical compounds are used in the manufacture of agricultural insecticides and weed killers, one of which, cacodylic acid (dimethyly arsenic acid) is quite commonly used by foresters in the United States. Some fungicides and wood preservations contain arsenic and so do some sheep and cattle dips. In the glass industry it is used to remove the green tint produced by iron oxide. Anti-fouling compounds for ships may contain arsenic and they are also used in dyes and soaps. Arsenic is added to some alloys in small amounts (0.3–0.5 per cent) to increase hardening and heat resistance and similar amounts added to molten lead make the metal harder and assist in the formation of truly spherical pellets of lead shot. A number of organic arsenical compounds are still in therapeutic use.

Arsenical pigments were once widely used, and they resulted in a considerable morbidity. Cupric arsenite (Scheele's green) enjoyed great popularity in the nineteenth century as a colouring for wallpaper and was capable of releasing dimethyl arsine through the action of a mould growing in the paste, which it is said could prove fatal. These compounds are seldom met nowadays.

Hazards of use: Industrial risks mainly result from the inhalation of the very light dust of the arsenical compound during handling processes, but some vapour may be encountered during the smelting and refining of ores.

Crop-sprayers are at risk from arsenic which comes into contact with the skin. They may also, of course, inhale the spray if not properly protected.

Metabolism: Inorganic arsenic compounds are absorbed by inhalation, ingestion and through the intact skin. Over 95 per cent of arsenic in the blood is bound to the protein of haemoglobin. It is stored in the tissues, and tends to accumulate in the muscles and liver, and to a lesser extent in the other viscera, and particularly in hair and nails. The affinity of arsenic for the protein in hair is the basis of forensic tests for detecting arsenical poisoning.

Excretion takes place predominantly through the kidney. In the urine arsenic is mainly in the organic, methylated form. The concentration of arsenic in the urine is a reasonable indication of the degree of exposure and is the most widely used form of biological monitoring.

Acute poisoning: Acute poisoning in industry is rare but when it is seen, it is the result of inhaling high concentrations of dust. The first symptoms are those of severe respiratory irritation with cough, inspiratory chest pain and dyspnoea. These early symptoms are followed by headache, vertigo and lassitude and those gastro-intestinal symptoms such as are seen after the ingestion of arsenic or its compounds.

Acute poisoning by ingestion is the more common presentation and is usually the result of arsenic administered for suicidal or homicidal purposes. If the dose is large enough, the victim may collapse and die within 20 minutes. More often, however, smaller doses are ingested which produce vomiting, diarrhoea, abdominal pain and muscle cramps. If the patient survives he usually has no sequelae although a few cases are known in which exfoliative dermatitis and peripheral neuropathy have developed.

Chronic poisoning: Chronic intoxication particularly affects the skin and is discussed in Chapter 6. Peripheral neuropathy appears in some cases and is usually accompanied by pain, burning and tenderness, and difficulty in walking. The presence of broad white striae on the finger nails (mees lines) is said to be diagnostic.

Gastro-intestinal symptoms, including nausea, vomiting and abdominal pain occur, but none is common.

Arsenic dust has a local action on the mucous membranes producing conjunctivitis, blepharitis, rhinitis, pharyngitis, laryngitis and bronchitis. Hoarseness may be a prominent symptom and painless perforation of the cartilaginous part of the nasal septum is sometimes observed. Arsenic dust in the glass industry produces a well-recognized rash on the skin. The carcinogenic action of arsenic is considered in Chapter 8.

Organic arsenic compounds

The organic arsenic compounds are powerful vesicants and lung irritants and exposure to these compounds is restricted to the chemists who synthesize them and to those who are concerned with their development as war gases. BAL. (British Anti-Lewisite), was developed specifically to counter the action of the arsenical war gas, Lewisite (chlorovinyl dichlorarsine). It is a dithiol compound, 2, 3,-dimercapto propanol, and owes its efficacy to the high affinity which arsenic has for sulphydryl (—SH) groups. BAL was later used in the treatment of lead and mercury poisoning on the basis of their known affinity for —SH groups, but it has now been largely replaced by EDTA and penicillamine.

Aluminium

Aluminium is very widely used both alone and alloyed with other metals in the manufacture of household utensils, laboratory equipment, cables and wires, packaging materials, foils and reflectors, and powder for use in paints.

Exposure to pure aluminium dust may produce a form of pulmonary fibrosis, the main feature of which is a rapidly progressive dyspnoea with cough and weight loss. The pathological changes are mainly confined to the upper zones and on chest X-ray are revealed as reticular or honeycomb markings. The lower lung fields may be emphysematous and spontaneous pneumothoraces occur.

The course of the disease is rapid and death may follow in as little as two years from the onset of symptoms although some improvement is to be expected if exposure is discontinued.

Nowadays, when aluminium powder is stamped out the surface is covered with stearates and in its protected form it is not hazardous. There is no hazard for health from the use of aluminium pots and pans in cooking.

Antimony

Antimony is used industrially in several metallurgical processes, in the ceramic and glass industries, as a pigment in paints, and in the rubber and plastics industries. Antimony compounds are also used in the manufacture of semi-conductors to 'dope' crystals in much the same way as arsine is used (see p. 93). Although it is known to be toxic, cases of poisoning usually arise from mishaps outside industry, often through overdosage with compounds such as potassium antimony tartarate (tartar emetic) used to treat schistosomiasis or from the preparation and storage of food in vessels with an antimony glaze.

The symptoms of acute poisoning are similar to those of acute arsenical poisoning although vomiting is more severe and continuous and accompanied by watery diarrhoea. Cardiac arrhythmias have been frequently noted as toxic manifestations of antimony poisoning and the mortality rate from this complication may be considerable. Mild jaundice has also been noted, whilst in a number of cases, a maculo-papular rash has been observed.

The antimony used in industry is frequently contaminated with arsenic and toxic symptoms noted in men handling antimony ores have often been attributed to the arsenic present. In some cases, however, it seems likely that antimony was producing adverse reactions in those exposed to dust and fume, including such symptoms as vomiting, diarrhoea, vertigo and headaches. Electrocardiographic changes have been reported in some workers, the most common being abnormalities of the T-wave. On the skin, antimony may produce punched out ulcers, 'antimony pocks' which usually appear on the forearms and are slow to heal.

Osmium

Osmium is not itself toxic, but osmium tetroxide, used as an histological stain, is irritant to the mucous membranes of the eyes, nose, pharynx and bronchus. In high concentrations it produces a constriction of the chest, an inability to breathe and, rarely, a fatal bronchiolitis. Osmium tetroxide vapour is so irritant that the risk of inhaling a lethal quantity is slight. Continued inhalation of small amounts, however, is said to predispose to bronchitis and chemical pneumonitis. Headache is some-times a feature of mild intoxication and characteristically, a halo is seen around light sources.

Platinum

Platinum salts give rise to a pronounced irritation of the nose and upper respiratory tract, which in turn produces a running nose and a cough. Platinum asthma is a common and important condition arising in those exposed to chloroplatinic acid or one of its salts and normally results only after prolonged exposure. This is not an invariable rule however. Skin lesions are also produced, consisting of a dry scaly dermatitis which cracks and bleeds. This combination of respiratory and dermatological disorders is sometimes called platinosis.

Platinum metal (in those who can afford it) may give rise to a contact dermatitis.

Selenium and Tellurium

These metalloids are chemically analogous. Selenium, being more soluble in body fluids is more toxic than tellurium and its compounds may produce dermatitis; selenium oxychloride is highly vesicant. Selenium fume has an intensely irritant effect on the eyes, nose and throat and also produces severe headaches. The chronic effects of selenium have been reported to include upper respiratory tract irritation, vague gastrointestinal disturbances and a smell of garlic on the breath; it may also induce liver damage in those heavily exposed. The smell of garlic (also produced by tellurium) is caused by the exhalation of the dimethyl compound formed by a detoxifying methylation reaction in the liver. The smell quickly disappears once exposure is discontinued and there is no treatment for it.

Tellurism is the name given to the syndrome which comprises dry mouth, dry skin, metallic taste, nausea, anorexia, somnolence and vomiting. Scaly pruritic skin lesions have also occurred after exposure to tellurium fumes.

Acute poisoning with selenium and tellurium is not known in industry. Fatalities have been caused by accidental exposure outside industry, however, and at autopsy the major findings have been haemorrhagic congestion of various organs with focal bleeding.

Silver

Although silver produces no constitutional symptoms, absorbed silver is precipitated in the tissues where it is fixed and becomes dissolved, producing either local or generalized argyria. Local argyria is more common, resulting from the impregnation of the skin with small particles of silver. These are converted first to silver albuminate and then to silver sulphide which produces discrete areas of grey-blue pigmentation. Local lesions may be found in the eyes, confined to the conjunctiva.

In the more rare generalized argyria, the uncovered areas of skin are a uniform dark, slate-grey colour. Affected men are known as 'blue men'. The finger-nails are chocolate brown and the buccal mucosa is grey or blue in colour. The covered parts of the skin are as a rule unaffected or at most only faintly pigmented. The conjunctiva are discoloured grey to deep brown and examination of the lens with a slit lamp shows a grey pigmentation of Decemet's membrane. There is usually no disturbance of vision.

In cases of generalized argyria which come to autopsy, silver granules can be found in the internal organs and in the mucosa of the respiratory tract. The granules are also seen in the internal elastic laminae of the arterioles, in the elastic fibres of connective tissue, in the connective tissue between myocardial fibrils, and in the basement membranes of sweat glands, renal tubule cells and the ependymal cells of the choroid plexus. The testes may appear black, but here as elsewhere, no interference with function is recorded as a result of the silver impregnation.

Thallium

Thallium is an extremely toxic substance, more toxic than lead, but less toxic than arsenic. Industrial poisoning is rare despite its great potential for harm: it is absorbed via every route, cutaneous, pulmonary and gastrointestinal. Excretion is slow and the metal is cumulative.

Acute poisoning is typified by vomiting, diarrhoea, colic, insomnia, joint pains, psychotic disturbances and an ascending paralysis which may be mistaken for the Guillain-Barré syndrome. Chronic poisoning is characterized by polyneuritis and loss of hair. Ocular lesions are common including retrobulbar neuritis, optic atrophy and lens opacities. Albuminuria is often noted. There is no treatment.

Tin

Exposure to inorganic tin compounds produces a benign pneumoconiosis referred to as stannosis. The pleura and lymph nodes are pigmented black. The radiological picture may be confused with silicosis (*q.v.*).

Organotin compounds are increasingly in use; the disubstituted compounds are used as stabilizers and catalysts in the plastic industry and the tri-substituted ones as fungicides and biocides.

In general, organotin compounds are strong irritants and skin burns and conjunctivitis may follow accidental splashing. They may also cause liver and kidney damage and they have haemolytic activity. The tri-substituted compounds are much more toxic than those which are bi-substituted; tri-ethyl tin is particularly neurotoxic and is capable of producing a toxic encephalopathy.

CHAPTER 3/INDUSTRIAL TOXICOLOGY
2: ORGANIC SOLVENTS

Many thousands of organic compounds are used in industry and large numbers of new compounds are introduced each year. Many of the organic compounds are used as solvents and hence exposure to solvents is widespread. As with the metals, it will be possible here to mention only the most important of the selection available, and a few general considerations of some of the metabolic and toxicological properties of solvents may be helpful in understanding what follows.

General considerations of
solvent metabolism and toxicology

Organic solvents—by which one simply means any compound used to carry another in solution—may be either fat or water soluble and they may undergo biotransformation in the body or circulate unchanged. Their solubility determines their distribution within the body. Fat soluble solvents tend to accumulate selectively in the organs rich in lipids, including the nervous system. Water soluble solvents, on the other hand, enter the body water compartment and have the potential to become much more widely distributed. All solvents are readily absorbed through the lung in their vapour phase, but fat soluble solvents may also be absorbed through the skin.

Solvents which are not biotransformed are excreted either in exhaled air or unchanged in the urine. From the solvents which are biotransformed (and these are the majority), metabolites appear in the urine and their rate of excretion may be used to monitor exposure at work. For all solvents, biological monitoring may also include estimations of the concentration of the unchanged compound in the exhaled air or in the blood.*

Just as with metals, interactions are important in determining the metabolic and toxic consequences of solvent exposure. Many organic

*It should be noted that it is more accurate to talk of biotransformation than detoxification when considering the metabolism of organic compounds, because in a number of cases, the daughter compounds are more toxic than their parents.

compounds interfere with the metabolism of others, mainly through competition for common pathways. Thus the rate of metabolism of two (or more) benzene analogues will be slower when given together than when administered separately; the co-administration of two chemically unrelated species such as trichloroethylene and benzene may also result in metabolic interference due to competition for co-factors.

One interesting interaction is that between ethanol and some solvents. The biotransformation of the benzene analogues, for example, follows a common pathway, the first step of which is an oxidation to form the alcohol derivative. This is followed by a reduction reaction brought about by alcohol dehydrogenase using NADP as co-factor. In acute experiments it can be shown that when alcohol is co-administered with a benzene analogue the biotransformation of the solvent is considerably delayed. Under experimental conditions, when the molar dose of ethanol far exceeds that of the solvent the ethanol is able to compete successfully for the enzyme and thus delay the biotransformation of the solvent. The solvent will be metabolized again when the relative solvent/ethanol concentrations are in favour of the solvent.

The effects of alcohol on solvent metabolism, however, are not as simple as acute exposure chamber studies would lead one to believe. Ethanol is an enzyme inducer and continuous exposure leads to an increase in the activity of the P-450 mixed function oxidazes which catalyse the initial oxidation of many solvents. Thus animals given ethanol over a long time may be able to biotransform solvents at a rate which is quicker than normal and there is also some suggestion that amongst men at work, consistently heavy drinkers get rid of solvents faster than their more abstemious colleagues.

So far as toxic effects are concerned, there is good reason to suppose that alcohol will add to any central nervous system effects induced by exposure to solvents but there is so far precious little evidence that psychotropic drugs interact with solvents. There is good evidence also that the neurotoxic effects of solvents is affected by co-exposure. For example, the weak neurotoxicity of a material such as methyl ethyl ketone may be enhanced by other solvents in a mixture whereas the neurotoxicity of n-hexane is diminished by co-administration of toluene.

The practical significance of these interactions becomes apparent when one realizes that exposures at work are often to mixtures of solvents rather than to single compounds and this must be taken into account when setting safety standards or devising programmes for biological monitoring.

AROMATIC SOLVENTS

Benzene

Uses: Benzene is the starting point for a great many synthetic processes in the chemical industry; it was formerly used on a grand scale as a solvent but its toxicity is such that it has been banned from general use if present in a concentration greater than 1 per cent in any solvent. It may be a component of motor fuel. In essential processes in this country it is used entirely in closed systems so that exposures are low. In less developed countries, however, benzene is used as a solvent in the manufacture of rubber or plastic shoes and in photogravure printing; exposures amongst those who use benzene for these purposes may be extremely high.

Hazards of use: Closed systems present little hazard and the only possibility of excessive exposure arises when the systems are maintained or repaired. Operators undertaking such work must be adequately equipped with protective clothing. Where benzene is used as a solvent there is an ever-present danger particularly if it is used in a poorly ventilated workshop.

Metabolism: Benzene is absorbed through the lungs and through the skin. It is lipid soluble and so accumulates in the fatty tissues which act as a reservoir. A large amount of absorbed benzene is exhaled unchanged but between 15–60 per cent is biotransformed. The biotransformation of benzene is complex but the preliminary step is oxidation to benzene epoxide which, like all epoxides is highly reactive and may combine with proteins or with nucleic acids. Benzene epoxide may undergo spontaneous transformation to phenol or it may be hydrated and reduced to catechol or condensed with glutathione to form mercapturic acid. The biological half life is about 12 hours.

Acute poisoning: This is the more uncommon form of poisoning encountered in industry and is due to accidental exposure to very high concentrations of vapour. The early symptoms include euphoria, giddiness, headache and vomiting. If the victim is not rescued from his exposure unconsciousness and death from respiratory failure may follow.

Chronic poisoning: Benzene is outstanding amongst the industrial poisons in having its principal effects on the bone marrow. There are usually no symptoms in the early stages of chronic intoxication and those which are present tend to be vague and nonspecific and do not correspond in any degree with the severity of the damage inflicted upon the bone marrow. Symptoms of tiredness, mild gastro-intestinal disturbance and giddiness are usually first noted and these are followed by haemorrhages from mucous membranes and the development of skin rashes. Anaemia is a common finding in workers with chronic benzene poisoning and this may be accompanied by macrocytosis and thrombocytopaenia. Myelocytes and nucleated red cells may be seen in the peripheral blood film and the red cells show basophilic stippling. Leucopaenia is a frequent finding, with a relative and absolute lymphopaenia. In the early stages the bone marrow may be hyperplastic but if exposure is not discontinued, a true aplastic anaemia may develop with the destruction of all the cellular elements. Aplastic anaemia is the most feared consequence of exposure to benzene and it is thought that the toxic agent is a metabolite which interferes with DNA synthesis; increased rates of chromosome aberrations are seen in workers exposed to benzene and in experimental animals.

Exposure to benzene is also associated with the development of acute leukaemia. Most cases are of the acute myeloblastic type but a few cases of erythroleukaemia have also been described. Leukaemia most often occurs in patients who already have a hypoplastic marrow and a history of heavy exposure is invariable. There may be an interval of several years between the end of last exposure and the development of the leukaemia. It should be noted in passing that not all authorities are convinced that benzene can cause leukaemia but the majority of opinion is against them.

Treatment: Patients with acute poisoning must be removed from exposure and respiratory support given where necessary; this is the case, of course, whatever solvent is involved. There are usually no serious late sequelae.

For those who develop aplastic anaemia or leukaemia following benzene exposure the prognosis is the same as in any other form of these diseases, that is, not outstandingly hopeful. On this account, all those who are exposed to benzene should have regular haematological examinations and those showing any abnormalities should be removed from exposure. Urinary phenol estimations are a useful adjunct to biological monitoring as they correlate reasonably well with exposure; with exposures at the current TLV of 10 ppm, urinary phenol concentrations at the end of the day would not be expected to exceed about 20 mgm/l.

Toluene

Uses: Toluene is one of the most widely used solvents in industry. It is found in paints, resins and glues, as a solvent for rubber and in photogravure printing. It is also an important raw material for synthetic reactions.

Hazards of use: All processes in which toluene are used should be properly ventilated in order to minimize exposure and care should be taken when handling drums to avoid spillage. Toluene is one of the solvents which is commonly sniffed and although sniffing seems to be mainly an out of work pastime, attention should be given to the identification of sniffers in the work force. At normal temperatures toluene gives off highly inflammable vapours and great care must be taken to minimize the risk of fire and explosion. If a vessel which has contained toluene is to be welded or cut with a flame all traces of vapour must be removed by purging.

Metabolism: Toluene is absorbed through the lung and, to a limited degree only, through the skin. Being lipid soluble it accumulates in fatty organs. The biological half life is 3–4 hours so that it is rapidly excreted once exposure is discontinued. Less than 10 per cent of an absorbed dose is exhaled unchanged, the remainder being biotransformed, mainly to hippuric acid (see Fig. 3.1); small amounts of *o*-crēsol and *p*-cresol are also formed.

Toluene → benzyl alcohol → benzaldehyde →
benzoic acid + glucuronic acid → hippuric acid

Fig. 3.1. Metabolism of toluene in man.

Toxic effects: All solvents have narcotic properties which many solvent workers experience from time to time. The concentration at which these properties manifest themselves obviously varies from solvent to solvent and their narcotic powers also differ; those which are most narcotic are, or have been, used as anaesthetics. Above about 1000 ppm, toluene causes vertigo and an intense headache, higher concentrations may induce coma. High concentrations are also hallucinogenic and it is for this reason that glues containing toluene are sniffed. At much lower concentrations, it is usual to find some evidence of undue tiredness, and vague feelings of ill health which have recovered by the start of the next working shift. Toluene does not depress the bone marrow and it is not notably hepatotoxic.

Toluene does not affect the peripheral nervous system and the evidence that prolonged exposure may induce organic brain damage is tenuous. Experience in this country would suggest that permanent neuropsychological sequelae are not a consequence of toluene exposure. In glue sniffers there have been very few reports of permanent damage and that which is most commonly reported is cerebellar degeneration. Some sudden deaths in glue sniffers have been ascribed to ventricular arrhythmias due to sensitization of the myocardium to circulating catecholamines but the cause is probably more complex than this since the technique used by glue sniffers frequently results in hypercapnia and acidosis.

Xylene

Uses: Xylene is much less commonly encountered than toluene but it is used as a thinner for paints and varnishes, in the synthesis of dyes and as an additive to aviation fuels. It is also used in histology laboratories as a solvent for paraffin.

Metabolism: Pulmonary retention of xylene is high, between 60–65 per cent of an inhaled dose being absorbed. It is also well absorbed through the skin and dermal absorption is a significant route of entry in industry. Virtually all the xylene which is absorbed is excreted in the form of metabolites, less than 5 per cent being exhaled unchanged. The route of biotransformation is similar to that of toluene with the formation of methylhippuric acid which appears in the urine (Fig. 3.2).

Xylene → methyl benzyl alcohol → methyl benzaldehyde → methyl benzoic acid + glucuronic acid → methyl hippuric acid

Fig. 3.2. Metabolism of xylene in man.

Poisoning: The symptoms of acute poisoning are similar to those of toluene poisoning but xylene is, in addition, an irritant with an unpleasant smell and workers may notice effects on the eyes and the upper respiratory tract. There is no well recognized symptom of chronic intoxication although it may cause an irritant dermatitis and some workers complain of a sweetish taste in the mouth. It is not hepatotoxic or neurotoxic.

Styrene

Uses: Styrene is a highly reactive compound because of the vinyl group which it has in its molecule, and it readily undergoes polymerization, oxidation, hydration or halogenation. It is common to add 3 per cent hydroquinone to styrene to inhibit its polymerization during storage or transport. Its principal uses are in the manufacture of polystyrene and of synthetic rubbers and it is used to carry the resin used in making glass reinforced plastics.

Metabolism: Styrene is avidly absorbed through the lungs and it is also readily absorbed through the skin. A small fraction only (< 5 per cent) is excreted unchanged and in man, the principal metabolic route leads to the formation of mandelic and phenylglyoxylic acids which are excreted in the urine. The biological half life of phenylglyoxylic acid in the urine is longer than that of mandelic acid and so is excreted for a longer time when exposure is discontinued. The first stage in the process is oxidation to form styrene oxide which is a highly reactive compound with mutagenic properties. It is for this reason that the carcinogenicity of styrene has been investigated. Styrene oxide is very short lived, however, and is rapidly reduced to styrene glycol (Fig. 3.3). In some animals mandelic acid is converted to benzyl alcohol with subsequent formation of hippuric acid which is the main breakdown product. Less than 1 per cent of the styrene absorbed is oxidized on the aromatic ring to form styrene 3,4 oxide which is then converted to vinylphenol; this is of academic rather than practical interest.

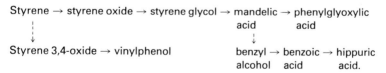

Styrene → styrene oxide → styrene glycol → mandelic → phenylglyoxylic
                                                acid   acid
  ↓   ↓
Styrene 3,4-oxide → vinylphenol   benzyl → benzoic → hippuric
                                         alcohol acid   acid.

Fig. 3.3. Metabolism of styrene in man.

Toxicity: Styrene has all the narcotic potential of other solvents and produces feelings of lassitude and vague ill health at the end of the day. In addition it has an irritant vapour which may affect the eyes, nose and upper respiratory tract and the skin. It also produces an unpleasant metallic taste in the mouth. It is not neurotoxic and not notably hepatotoxic although there are some reports of elevated levels of bile acids in the blood of solvent workers with otherwise normal liver function; the significance of these findings waits to be clarified. There are some largely anecdotal accounts that styrene workers are unusually short-tempered and argumentative late in a day on which they have been heavily exposed but formal proof of this assertion is wanting.

Ethylbenzene: This compound is chemically similar to styrene (except that it lacks the vinyl group) and is used in the manufacture of styrene and cellulose acetate; it has virtually the same metabolic pathway as styrene, being broken down to mandelic and phenylglyoxylic acids. Lacking the reactive double bond, it is less irritant that styrene but is more volatile and so more likely to produce narcotic symptoms.

CHLORINATED HYDROCARBONS

The chlorinated hydrocarbons are noninflammable, noncombustible and nonexplosive and thus find extensive use through industry as degreasing agents, rubber and plastic solvents, paint solvents, refrigerants and dry cleaning fluids and some are used as fungicides and in fire extinguishers.

The introduction of chlorine into a hydrocarbon molecule generally enhances its toxicity and this toxicity increases with increasing molecular weight. As a rule the toxicity of chlorinated hydrocarbons is a function of the instability of the halogen ion and the more volatile the compound, the greater its toxicity.

Although they do not combust, at high temperatures, halogenated hydrocarbons are decomposed in the presence of air to produce highly toxic compounds including the free halide, hydrogen halides and carbonyl halides of which phosgene ($COCl_2$) is a particularly unpleasant example.

Carbon tetrachloride

Uses: Carbon tetrachloride is used in the production of freons but it was formerly much used as a solvent, as a fumigant, in fire extinguishers and as a dry cleaning agent for both domestic and industrial use. Because of its high toxicity, it has been superseded where possible by other compounds.

Metabolism: Carbon tetrachloride is readily absorbed through the lungs and it concentrates in the fatty tissues. About half of an absorbed dose is excreted unchanged in exhaled air and about 5 per cent is eliminated as carbon dioxide. The remainder is excreted in the urine but the precise nature of the metabolite (or metabolites) has not been determined. Carbon tetrachloride is also metabolized by ribosomal enzymes to the highly reactive CCl_3 radical through a series of hydroxylation reactions. This radical is the putative toxic agent and only those cells which contain the appropriate enzyme system are sensitive to its effects.

The toxic effects of carbon tetrachloride are enhanced by enzyme inducers such as phenobarbitone and alcohol; in addition, alcohol enhances the uptake of carbon tetrachloride from the gut.

Poisoning: In rapidly fatal cases of carbon tetrachloride poisoning, the narcotic effect produces unconsciousness which is preceded by signs of central nervous system disturbance. Such cases are extemely rare now. In severe but not immediately fatal cases, the symptoms are predomin-antly those due to liver or renal damage. Usually renal symptoms are more striking than hepatic symptoms. Initially the patient will complain of a persistent headache, nausea and vomiting, colic and diarrhoea, and hepatic tenderness. Signs of renal or hepatic damage appear after a variable latent interval. Renal signs include oliguria with albumin, casts and red cells in the urine and a raised blood urea. Total anuria may point to a fatal outcome. Hepatic damage is indicated by the development of jaundice and alterations in liver function tests. Cardiac arrhythmias and ventricular fibrillation have also been recorded. Pathological changes include centrilobular necrosis and fatty degeneration in the liver and proximal tubular necrosis in the kidney.

Carbon tetrachloride is a highly potent experimental carcinogen and it has been widely used to induce hepatic tumours in rats and mice. There is no evidence that it has this effect in man.

Tetrachloroethane

Uses: Tetrachloroethane is now used only as an intermediate in the manufacture of tetrachloroethylene and trichloroethylene. It was formerly used to a much greater extent but on account of its great toxicity, it has been replaced by other solvents.

Metabolism: It is absorbed through the lung and skin and is eliminated slowly from the body. Its metabolism is complex; some is converted to trichloroethylene and dichloroacetaldehyde which are subsequently broken down to trichloroethanol and trichloroacetic acid, and glyoxalic acid and glycine respectively. Tetrachloroethane is itself broken down to form trichloroacetic acid and oxalic acid.

Poisoning: Tetrachloroethane is the most toxic of the chlorinated hydrocarbons; it has a smell which resembles that of chloroform but it has two or three times the narcotic effect of chloroform. There are two principal syndromes of tetrachloroethane poisoning, the neurological and the hepatic. A toxic polyneuropathy was first noted amongst girls working to make artificial pearls and in other workers, signs of central nervous system effects have been noted, including tremor, vertigo and headaches. Four stages in the hepatic syndrome have been described, the end result being toxic jaundice and death.

1,1,1-Trichloroethane (methyl chloroform)

Uses: Trichloroethane is one of the most widely used solvents especially for the degreasing of metal. It is inflammable and does not support combustion but at 260°C it decomposes to form hydrochloric acid and traces of phosgene.

Metabolism: Trichloroethane is rapidly absorbed through the lung and to a small extent through the skin. It is mainly excreted unchanged in expired air, less than 10 per cent being metabolized. Some of that which is metabolized is converted to carbon dioxide but the majority is converted to trichloroethanol.

Poisoning: There are no serious ill effects following exposure to trichloroethane at the concentrations usual in industry; contact with the skin will produce a mild irritant dermatitis (as will all degreasing agents) and conjunctivitis is to be expected if a splash gets in the eyes. It has the usual narcotic effects at high concentrations and was used briefly as an anaesthetic with no accounts of hepatic or renal damage or of cardiac dysfunction.

A few fatalities have occurred following exposure to extremely high concentrations usually as the result of using the solvent in a confined space so that an anaesthetic concentration was generated. Death resulted from respiratory depression or cardiac arrhythmia.

Trichloroethylene

Uses: Trichloroethylene is non-explosive, non-inflammable, very volatile and cheap so that it comes as no surprise to find it is one of the most successful solvents ever put on the market. It is still widely used as a degreasing agent and for organic synthesis in the chemical industry. At one time it was extensively used as a dry cleaning agent and as a refrigerant but it has generally been replaced by other solvents for these purposes. It is still used on a limited scale as an anaesthetic in obstetric practice.

Metabolism: Trichloroethylene is rapidly absorbed from the lungs, the retention rate ranging from 45–75 per cent; it can also penetrate the skin. Very little is eliminated unchanged on the breath, the majority being broken down to trichloroethanol and trichloroacetic acid (see Fig. 3.4).

Trichloroethylene → trichloroacetaldehyde → chloral hydrate → trichloroethanol + trichloroacetic acid

Fig. 3.4. Metabolism of trichloroethylene in man.

The formation of trichloroethanol from chloral hydrate is the result of a rapid reduction whereas trichloroacetic acid is formed by a slow oxidation. The half lives of the two compounds differs; for trichloroacetic acid it is between 70–100 hours because it binds to plasma proteins, whereas for trichloroethanol the half life is only 10–15 hours. There appears to be a sex difference in the metabolism of trichloroethylene. In men, the excretion of trichloroethanol is greater than in women whereas the converse is true for trichloroacetic acid.

Poisoning: Trichloroethylene is a powerful narcotic which, of course, makes it a good anaesthetic. It also produces a pleasant euphoria which may lead to addiction. Mild narcotic effects will be noted following exposures to moderately high concentrations but these are short lasting and of no long term consequence. It is not nearly as hepatotoxic as chloroform, carbon tetrachloride or tetrachloroethane, but liver damage has been reported in a number of fatal cases due to acute poisoning.

There is some debate as to whether a syndrome of chronic poisoning really exists. Some authorities report that lassitude, giddiness, irritability, headache and gastro-intestinal disturbances follow repeated exposures and that they may persist for several weeks or months after the cessation of exposure. There is not much support for this view in this country.

Although trichloroethylene does not cause peripheral neuropathy, there have been a few undoubted cases of cranial nerve damage both following anaesthetic use and exposure at work. The Vth, VIth, VIIIth, IXth and XIIth cranial nerves may all be affected but the Vth suffers most; in a fatal case, gross degeneration of the nerve and its nuclei was found at autopsy. The proximate toxic substance is not known with certainty but is thought to be dichloroacetylene.

Trichloroethylene is one of the solvents most likely to account for the so-called sudden death syndrome. Characteristically, death occurs in a young person who has been heavily exposed to the solvent following some sudden exertion such as running up stairs. Death is thought to be due to ventricular fibrillation brought about by sensitization of the myocardium to catecholamines. The effect can be induced in experimental animals and prevented by the co-administration of calcium.

One interesting effect of trichloroethylene is to produce a facial vasodilation in response to drinking alcohol; the effect is known as degreasers' flush, a syndrome much favoured by examiners. The vasodilation is thought to be brought about by circulating trichloroacetaldehyde, the metabolism of which is inhibited by alcohol.

Tetrachloroethylene (perchloroethylene)

Uses: Tetrachloroethylene has replaced trichloroethylene to a large extent as a dry-cleaning fluid and as a degreasing agent.

Metabolism: The vapour is absorbed through the lungs and skin absorption occurs following contact with the liquid. It is stored for long periods in fatty tissues and there tends to be an accumulation of the solvent with repeated exposures. The solvent is released slowly from fat and this dictates the rate of elimination. Almost no tetrachloroethylene is metabolized and it is mainly excreted through the lung unchanged; the 3 per cent or so which is broken down, is excreted in the urine as trichloroacetic acid.

Poisoning: Apart from the usual narcotic effects, tetrachloroethylene has few untoward characteristics. In common with most other chlorinated hydrocarbon solvents, it has been found to be teratogenic to the chick by Russian workers; there are no indications that it is teratogenic to man.

Methylene chloride (dichloromethane)

Uses: Methylene chloride is a highly volatile solvent used in the manufacture of cellulose acetate film and it is a component of some paint strippers.

Metabolism: This solvent is absorbed through the lungs and probably through the skin. Methylene chloride is metabolized predominantly to carbon dioxide but a substantial proportion (about a third) is converted to carbon monoxide which combines with haemoglobin to form carboxyhaemoglobin. An 8 hour exposure to about 150 ppm of methylene chloride produces an equivalent amount of carboxyhaemoglobin as exposure to exposure to 35 ppm of carbon monoxide for the same time; in both cases the COHb level increases to about 5 per cent. For an equivalent exposure, smokers will have a greater COHb concentration than non-smokers.

Poisoning: Methylene chloride has—as you should by now expect —narcotic properties against which a worker ought to be able to protect himself for, at about 300 ppm, a sweet smell can be detected and this will alert the man to the fact that he is being exposed above the TLV. The discovery that methylene chloride was converted to carbon monoxide led to much speculation about the likelihood that exposure might cause cardiovascular or cerebrovascular disease. There have indeed been a small number of case reports of both occurring in men who have been unusually heavily exposed but there is no evidence to suggest that at the levels commonly encountered in industry, there is any increased risk of vascular disease.

Irritation of the skin and eyes may follow direct contact, and severe chemical burns have been found in one case of a man who was overcome by fumes and remained in contact with the liquid for several minutes.

OTHER SOLVENTS

Carbon disulphide

Uses: Carbon disulphide has a long and inglorious part to play in the history of occupational medicine. It was introduced into use in the 1850s as a rubber solvent and it was also used in the manufacture of matches in which process it acted as the solvent for phosphorus. Far and away the most important use of carbon disulphide now is in the production of

Chapter 3

viscose rayon fibres. Carbon disulphide is introduced into the process during xanthation of the alkali cellulose; sodium cellulose xanthate is formed which is dissolved in caustic soda to form viscose which can be spun into fibres or cast into cellophane. The xanthation process is enclosed so as to minimize exposure but carbon disulphide is liberated during all the spinning and casting processes and whenever the fibres break or are cut. Hydrogen sulphide is emitted at the same time.

Metabolism: Inhalation is the main route of entry but skin absorption also occurs. Between 70–90 per cent is metabolized, the remainder being excreted unchanged through the lungs. The compound is extremely active and has a high affinity for organic ligands and binds to amino acids, peptides and proteins in blood and tissues. Its metabolic pathways have not been worked out fully but it is known that a number of sulphur compounds appear in the urine including thiourea, mercaptothiazolinone and 2-thio-thiazolidine-4-carboxylic acid (mercifully shortened to TTCA).

Poisoning: Carbon disulphide is a multi-system poison and many toxic effects have been described. The most important are the neurological and cardiovascular effects but in addition it is a skin irritant, it may induce gastro-intestinal disorders, and it has been shown to cause abnormalities in thyroid and adreno-cortical function. It may also, of course, induce acute narcosis.

Neurological effects: Both the central and the peripheral nervous systems may be affected. Exposure to high concentrations of carbon disulphide may induce a toxic organic psychosis which was first recognized in Paris in the 1850s by August Delpech amongst the workers engaged in the cold vulcanization of rubber. The symptoms include extreme irritability, uncontrollable anger, insomnia, terrifying nightmares, loss of memory, delirium and headache. Later the patient may become depressed and paranoid and is at great danger of taking his own life. Clinically, it may be possible to detect both diffuse and focal neurological signs. The picture may be further complicated by the appearance of typical Parkinsonian features. The pathological correlates of this psychopathy are not clear; it has been suggested that it may be due to disturbances in the cerebral circulation, to the binding of free sulphur to neurofilaments, which interferes with normal axonal function, to the inhibition of dopamine-β-hydroxylase, or to disturbances in vitamin B_6 metabolism. Such a plethora of explanations suggests that none is sufficient fully to explain the condition.

The florid symptoms seen in the early days of carbon disulphide use are not encountered nowadays, indeed it would be a positive disgrace if they were. However, carbon disulphide is about the only solvent for which there is good evidence for sub-clinical neuropsychological effects. Carbon disulphide workers have a higher prevalence of abnormal EEGs than control subjects and they also perform less well in psychological tests than controls.

In the peripheral nervous system, carbon disulphide produces a mixed neuropathy which is pathologically identical with that produced by n-hexane and methyl-butyl-ketone (MBK). Nerve conduction velocities are slowed and this is an early indication of axonal damage; the conduction velocities return to normal if exposure is discontinued. The cardinal pathological sign is the appearance of swellings within the axon. These swellings first appear proximal to the node of Ranvier and the myelin overlying the swelling is absent or considerably thinned. (It is this which accounts for the slowing in nerve conduction.) Under the electron microscope it can be seen that the axonal swellings are due to the accumulation of 10 nm microfilaments and other intracellular organelles. This accumulation of debris interferes with the normal flow of material along the axon and the distal ends of the nerve fibres begin to die back. Similar changes can be seen within the brain stem. In carbon disulphide neuropathy the toxic agent is thought to be the carbon disulphide itself but it is not clear how it causes the neurofilamentous accumulations. It may be because it has a high affinity for —SH groups and is thus able to inhibit enzyme function or it may be that it is able to induce cross-linkage between proteins in the neurofilaments. Once exposure is discontinued there is a slow return to normal.

Cardiovascular effects: Carbon disulphide induces sclerotic changes in the arterial system the clinical effects of which depend upon the vessels most affected. Renal changes have been reported following unusually heavy exposure and cerebral arteriosclerosis has been postulated as causing some of the CNS effects. Perhaps the most significant effects, however, are those on the coronary arteries, and it has become clear in recent years that long term exposure to carbon disulphide is associated with a greatly increased prevalence of ischaemic heart disease, up to as much as five times greater than in a control population. When exposure is controlled it can be shown that the risk returns towards normal again.

Susceptibility to carbon disulphide: The compound tetraethylthiuram disulphide (TETD, Disulphiram, Antabuse) contains two CS_2 groups in its molecule and is broken down to diethyldithiocarbamate (DDC). The rate at which DDC appears in the urine after a dose of TETD is a measure of the subject's ability to handle sulphur-containing compounds and it has been suggested that susceptibility to carbon disulphide poisoning is inversely related to the amount of DDC excreted. It has been further suggested that prospective carbon disulphide workers should all undergo this test and only accepted if their excretion of DDC is in excess of 150 mg/g creatinine within 4 hours of a dose of 0.5 g of TETD.

n-Hexane and methyl-butyl ketone

It is appropriate to consider these solvents together since their metabolism and their toxic effects are similar.

Uses: n-Hexane is widely used as a solvent in glues and adhesives and in paints and dyes. MBK, and the other commonly used ketones, is used as a solvent for dyes, resins, gums, tars, waxes and fats and as an extractant in a range of synthetic processes.

Metabolism: n-Hexane is mainly taken up through the lungs and only about 15 per cent is retained. Skin absorption is extremely poor. MBK, by contrast, is readily absorbed by any route. The biotransformation of these compounds is inter-connected and both produce a toxic metabolite, 2,5-hexanedione (see Fig. 3.5.).

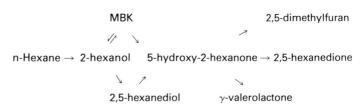

Fig. 3.5. Metabolism of n-hexane and methyl-butyl ketone (MBK) in man.

Poisoning: The principal toxic effect of these compounds is the production of a filamentous peripheral neuropathy similar to that produced by carbon disulphide. Both motor and sensory disturbances are noted but there is no interference with higher cerebral function. The proximate toxic agent is the common metabolite 2,5-hexanedione and it is the γ-diketone spacing in the molecule which is essential for its toxic effect.

Neither methyl ethyl ketone (MEK) nor methyl isobutyl ketone (MiBK) is neurotoxic since neither is metabolized to a compound containing the γ-diketone spacing within its molecule. It is of interest, however, that both MEK and MiBK are thought to be able to enhance the neurotoxicity of MBK so that solvents containing mixtures of ketones may be more neurotoxic than at first supposed.

The mechanism whereby 2,5-hexanedione induces the striking changes in the neurones is not clear. *In vitro*, it can be shown to inhibit some of the enzymes involved in the glycolytic pathway and it may also produce crosslinking of the neurofilaments by forming Schiff bases with amino groups.

Acetone

Acetone is one of the most safe of all solvents although it should not be forgotten that it is highly flammable and explosive. It is water soluble and enters the body mainly through inhalation. It appears unchanged in exhaled air and in the urine; it is also metabolized to formic acid.

Glycols and their derivatives

The glycols that are used commercially are colourless liquids which contain two hydroxyl groups per molecule which makes them chemically active and important as intermediates in synthetic processes. They are also completely water soluble and they are widely used as solvents for resins, lacquers, paints, dyes and inks. They are also used as antifreeze agents. The two in most common use are ethylene glycol and diethylene glycol.

Metabolism: Both compounds have a low volatility and inhalation is not an important route of entry and neither penetrates the skin. They are absorbed from the gut, however, and biotransformed to oxalic acid by alcohol dehydrogenase.

Poisoning: In normal use, neither of these compounds presents a serious hazard to health. If large quantities are ingested, however, either with the deliberate intention of self harm or in mistake for ethanol, there may be a deposition of calcium oxalate crystals within the renal tubules. Acute tubular necrosis and anuria will quickly follow and the patient will die unless treated promptly. Since ethanol is a better substrate than ethylene glycol for alcohol dehydrogenase, it is often advocated that patients with ethylene glycol poisoning should be given ethanol in order to slow down the breakdown of the glycol; haemodialysis should also form part of an effective treatment regime.

Glycol ethers

The glycol ethers are a large group of over 30 compounds. They are more volatile than the parent compounds and are miscible with water and most organic compounds and they are thus widely used as dispersants in industry. They are used as solvents for resins, paints and inks and they are important solvents for cellulose ester and mitrocellulose. The most important of the group are ethylene glycol monomethyl ether (methyl cellosolve), ethylene glycol monoethyl ether (cellosolve) and ethylene glycol iso-propyl ether, ethylene glycol n-butyl ether and propylene glycol monomethyl ether. Fortunately, these compounds are generally referred to by their abbreviated form, EGME, EGEE, EGiPE, EGBE and PGME.

Metabolism: Since they are more volatile than their parent compounds all the glycol ethers are inhaled through the lung and they may also be absorbed through the skin. Their subsequent metabolism largely determines their toxicity. Those compounds which contain a primary alcohol are good substrates for ADH and are oxidized to the corresponding alkoxyacids which have a high toxicity. Thus, methoxyacetic acid is formed from EGME, butoxyacetic acid is formed from EGBE and, by analogy, one would expect ethyoxyacetic acid to be formed from EGEE. From EGiPE, isopropoxyacetic acid has been recovered in dogs and rats. As an alternative route, the ether linkage may be cleaved with the production of oxalic acid and carbon dioxide; about 14 per cent of the total dose may be excreted as CO_2. By contrast, PGME is not a good substrate for ADH since it contains a secondary alcohol group and so it is mainly broken down to carbon dioxide and to PGME-glucuronide and sulphates which appear in the urine; these compounds account for 10–20 per cent of the total metabolites.

Poisoning: The glycol ethers and the ethylene derivatives are more toxic than the propylene derivatives and EGME is probably the most toxic of the group in common use. During the early days of its use, it was found to cause a toxic encephalopathy which is not seen under present conditions of use. It also affected the bone marrow, causing anaemia and the appearance of immature leucocytes in the peripheral blood. EGBE has been found to cause a haemolytic anaemia in animals but this does not seem to be the case in man. The isopropyl and n-propyl glycol ethers may, in addition, cause liver and kidney damage. Splashes into the eye of any of the ethylene glycol ethers cause an irritant conjunctivitis with corneal clouding which may last for several days. Splashes of PGME cause a mild irritation only.

Some of the ethylene glycol ethers have been shown to be both fetotoxic and teratogenic and to cause testicular changes in animals with alterions in sperm morphology. The degree of toxicity to the reproductive system is inversely related to the size of the alkoxy group—as are the effects on the bone marrow. Thus, the order of toxicity is EGME > EGEE > EGBE. It may be noted that the reverse is the case so far as haemolytic effects are concerned.

The reproductive effects of glycol ethers have been noted in several species of animals but there is no good evidence for their occurrence in man. Nevertheless, there is now a trend away from the use of the ethylene glycol ethers in favour of PGME wherever possible; PGME has no teratogenic effects, it exerts only weak fetotoxicity at high doses and it has no effects on the testis.

Dioxane

Dioxane, diethylene ether, is a ring compound, and has been in use for over half a century. It is a solvent for waxes, fat, greases and mineral oils and a cellulose and nitrocellulose solvent. At room temperatures liquid dioxane can produce explosive air/vapour mixtures.

Metabolism: Dioxane is volatile and well absorbed through the lungs and probably also through the skin. Its main metabolic by-product is β-hydroxyethoxyacetic acid and almost none of an absorbed dose escapes biotransformation.

Poisoning: The vapour has the expected narcotic effect in excess and it also causes irritation of the eyes, nose and throat at concentrations in the range 200–300 ppm. Liver and kidney damage may follow excessive exposures and in fatal cases in which death resulted from renal failure, hepatic enlargement and haemorrhagic kidneys have been noted at autopsy. Dioxane produces tumours in experimental animals but such epidemiological studies as have been carried out on populations exposed at work have not demonstrated any excess risk.

White spirit

White spirit is one of the most commonly used of all solvents; in the USA it is also known as Stoddard solvent. It is a mongrel of a solvent containing many straight and branched paraffins and aromatic hydrocarbons; the aliphatic/aromatic ratio is generally about 4:1 but variations are common. White spirit is an important paint solvent and few home decorators can fail to have noted some of its effects. The metabolism of white spirit is complex. The major components will tend to be broken down in the normal way but the presence of so many other—often related—compounds will produce interactions, the degree of which cannot always be accurately predicted. White spirit has a vapour which has an unpleasant smell and which is mildly irritant; after a few minutes exposure, however, olfactory fatigue occurs and the smell is not noted. It may cause mild conjunctivitis and painters will generally admit to feelings of tiredness and general ill health which are greater than those experienced by other workers. In the Scandinavian countries there is a strong belief that exposure to white spirit may cause presenile dementia and in Finland and Denmark this is now a compensatable disease. In the UK no evidence has yet been found to suggest that exposure to white spirit causes any irreversible neuropsychological effects.

CHAPTER 4/INDUSTRIAL TOXICOLOGY 3: MISCELLANEOUS ORGANIC COMPOUNDS

Vinyl chloride

Vinyl chloride is a colourless gas which is used in the synthesis of polyvinyl chloride (PVC) a plastic without which modern life is almost unthinkable. It is flammable and when mixed with air in proportions between 4 and 22 per cent by volume is explosive.

Metabolism: The gas is rapidly absorbed through the lung and it also passes through the skin. It is quickly eliminated, either unchanged or as metabolites in the urine. The first step in its metabolism is oxidation to chloroethylene oxide which spontaneously rearranges to form chloro-acetaldehyde. This compound may be further oxidized to form mono-chloroacetic acid. The main urinary metabolites are hydroxyethyl cysteine, carboxyethyl cysteine, monochloroacetic acid and thiodiglycolic acid.

Poisoning: Acute effects such as a feeling of elation followed by lethargy are well recognized; at concentrations above 10,000 vertigo may be noted whilst hearing and vision are impaired when the concentration is greater than 16,000 ppm; loss of consciousness occurs with concentrations in excess of 70,000 ppm.

Constant exposure to high concentrations of the vapour may give rise to a chronic condition which is known as vinyl chloride disease. The major components of this syndrome are Raynaud's phenomenon, skin changes akin to scleroderma, acro-osteolysis, hepato-splenal fibrosis and haemangiosarcoma of the liver.

The Raynaud's phenomenon is caused by diffuse degenerative changes in the small blood vessels leading to occlusion of the capillaries and arterioles. Complete obliteration of the palmar arch may sometimes be noted at angiography. In association with the Raynaud's phenomenon, the skin of the hands and forearms may be inelastic and thinned; occasionally skin on other parts of the body may also be affected. The acro-osteolysis generally localized to the distal phalanges of the hands and is due to an aseptic necrosis caused by ischaemia. The bony changes

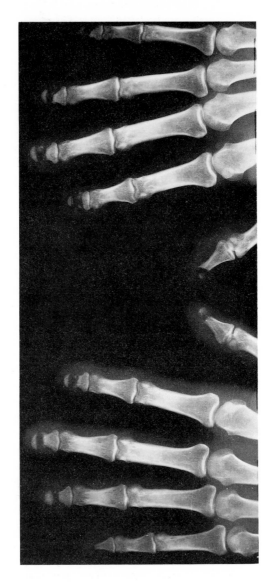

Fig. 4.1. Radiography showing the changes of acro–osteolysis in the fingers of both hands.

(Fig. 4.1) may progress to produce a transverse defect which subsequently heals to give a blunt, wide phalanx. Re-calcification may occur once exposure is discontinued.

The liver is affected in all cases of VCM poisoning. The liver may become enlarged but liver function tests are usually normal. If exposure is not discontinued at this stage, hepato-splenal fibrosis may supervene. There may be some elevation of transaminase levels but the diagnosis can be made only with an adequate liver biopsy. The parenchymal cells show relatively little change; a few swollen cells may be seen and some may be necrotic but fibrotic tissue can be seen in the portal spaces and extending between the parenchymal cells. When exposure is discontinued the hepatosplenomegaly and the parenchymal changes reverse but the fibrosis may deteriorate further.

The most serious of the components of vinyl chloride disease is angiosarcoma of the liver; this is rare and confined to men with extremely high exposures and one would not expect to see it in future with the advent of much more rigorous control limits.

It is clear from this account that vinyl chloride disease is a multi-system disorder, most likely with an immunological basis. Workers exposed to VCM have been found to have circulating immune complexes and immunofluorescent studies have shown that these complexes are deposited on the vascular endothelium. Other features which suggest that workers exposed to VCM suffer from an immune complex disorder include the finding of hyperimmunoglobulinaemia, cryoglobulinaemia together with *in vivo* complement activation via the classical pathway.

Acrylamide

Uses: Acrylamide is another vinyl monomer which will readily undergo polymerization and co-polymerization. It is used in the manufacture of flocculators which are substances which aid the separation of suspended solids from aqueous systems. As such they are useful in mining, soil stabilization and in the disposal of industrial wastes. Acrylamide is used also in the manufacture of paper, adhesives, fibres, dyes, pigments and leather substitutes and in the preparation of plastics and rubber.

Hazards of use: Only the monomer is toxic. Any process involving the handling of the monomer is potentially hazardous and workers should wear protective clothing to avoid getting it into contact with the skin.

Metabolism: Acrylamide may be absorbed by inhalation, ingestion or through the skin, but the last seems to be the most common path of entry. The fate of the substance in the body does not seem to have been reported.

Poisoning: The most serious effects are on the nervous system and two distinct lesions are produced, a peripheral neuropathy and a disturbance in the midbrain. Patients complain mainly of numbness and paraesthesiae in both upper and lower limbs with marked weakness, especially in the legs. Reflexes may be diminished or absent and there may be wasting of the muscles. Patients often have difficulty with their balance and they may be found to have an absence of vibration sense and a positive Romberg sign. In some the speech is slurred. Tiredness and lethargy are common, and there may be, in addition, generalized tremors, weight loss and impairment of bladder function. Increased sweating of the hands and feet are also noted. The palms may be erythematous, with peeling skin.

The condition invariably improves once exposure has been discontinued although the time required for the signs and symptoms to abate is variable. As with other industrial toxins, simple protective measures will safeguard those handling the monomer.

The substance has what has been called an anamnestic effect. That is to say, if acrylamide is administered to an animal which has recovered from the effects of acute intoxication, then the same symptoms will be produced by a lower dose of the drug. For this reason, men who have shown signs of intoxication are best not re-exposed.

Nitro and amino derivatives of benzene

The most important of these compounds are nitrobenzene, dinitrobenzene (DNB), trinitro toluene (TNT), aniline, dinitrophenol and dinitroortho cresol (DNOC).

Uses: These nitro and amino derivatives of benzene are intermediates used in the synthesis of more complex, but less toxic, molecules, the majority of which are used as dyes or explosives.

Hazards of use: All these substances can be absorbed through the skin and the lungs and the hazards associated with their use is dependent to a large extent on their physical state and their volatility. For this reason, aniline and nitrobenzene, which are bitter liquids, are regarded as more toxic than the solid DNB and TNT.

Metabolism: Absorption is possible through the lungs, the skin and the gastro-intestinal tract, but the first two routes are of greatest significance to industrial toxicology. Phenol derivatives are excreted in the urine, although DNB and TNT are also excreted unchanged.

Being lipid soluble, fatty tissues contain higher concentrations than do other tissues.

In the urine they are excreted mainly as phenol or nitro derivatives although DNB and TNT may be present unchanged.

Poisoning: All these compounds are capable of producing anaemia and toxic jaundice in varying degrees. The metabolites, notably p-amino phenol, oxidize the ferrous iron in haemoglobin to the ferric state forming methaemoglobin which binds oxygen much more firmly than does haemoglobin and some degree of tissue anoxia results, depending on the concentration in the blood. Methaemoglobin has a dark colour and when present in concentrations in excess of about 3 gm/100 ml produces a blue-grey discoloration of the skin sometimes referred to as 'toxic cyanosis'. This discoloration is most noticeable on the cheeks, ears, nose and finger-nails. The term anilism is applied to cases in which methaemoglobinaemia results from exposure to this class of chemicals and workers sometimes refer to themselves as being blued up.

The methaemoglobinaemia is accompanied by morphological changes in the circulating red cells. Examination of a peripheral blood film shows the presence of polychromasia, punctate basophilia and red cells containing Heinz bodies. Some of the amino-compounds have an irritant on the bladder producing a haemorrhage cystitis. Bladder cancer in workers handling these compounds is discussed further in Chapter 8.

Nitrobenzene: Nitrobenzene is an oily liquid known commercially as oil of mirbane. Acute poisoning most often follows the absorption of large amounts through the skin after the working clothes have become accidentally splashed. The symptoms of acute poisoning include fatigue, headache, vomiting and vertigo. In serious cases, unconsciousness supervenes and there are signs of circulatory collapse. The respiratory rate is first quickened, but slows if the patient becomes unconscious. The characteristic cyanosis is present and pronounced anaemia may follow. By about the third day jaundice and splenomegaly are noted on clinical examination.

The symptoms of acute poisoning may persist for many days and they may later be replaced or augmented by signs and symptoms due to excessive blood destruction. There are no late sequelae in those who survive.

Chronic poisoning follows long-term exposure to low concentrations and anaemia is the leading feature, with or without a mild haemolytic jaundice and albuminuria. Cyanosis, if present at all, is slight. Fatigue, headache, loss of appetite and cachexia are all found as a result of exposure and there may be erythema of exposed skin. Recovery may take several weeks and may not be complete.

Dinitrobenzene: DNB is a solid which is well absorbed through the skin. It is less toxic than nitrobenzene. Acute poisoning is manifested by the rapid onset of headache, vertigo and vomiting, and then by exhaustion, numbness in the legs and a staggering gait. The patient may become unconscious and cyanosed and death may result from central respiratory paralysis. In those who survive, the cyanosis exhaustion and vertigo are likely to persist for several days or weeks.

Chronic poisoning gives rise to weakness, fatigue, headaches and vomiting, and evening fever. Cyanosis and pallor are usually present. The usual blood changes will be found and albuminuria and porphyrinuria are occasionally present.

In many cases, those exposed to DNB become increasingly sensitive to its effects, so that the time interval between exposure and the development of cyanosis shortens. Acute exacerbations of symptoms has been known to occur following exposure to sunlight and after drinking alcohol. In each case, this is due to the liberation of DNB from fatty tissues in which it has been stored.

Trinitrotoluene: The skin is the important portal of entry for this solid material and absorption is greater in hot weather since TNT dust on the skin is dissolved in sweat. It is often used mixed with oxygen donors such as ammonium nitrate (amatol, ammonal) and barium nitrate (baratol).

Cyanosis and the usual blood changes indicate poisoning and in addition the hands and feet are sometimes stained orange. Symptoms of intoxication include a very irritant dermatitis and toxic gastritis. The patient has anorexia, nausea and vomiting and is constipated. The liver is usually enlarged and tender and the level of urinary coproporphyrin excretion is raised.

Treatment should be given in hospital. The skin must be thoroughly washed down with ether until there is no longer a pink reaction with alkaline ether. Recovery is usually complete but patients with toxic gastritis should not be re-exposed.

Toxic jaundice following exposure to TNT is rare but since it has a mortality rate of 30 per cent it is to be taken very seriously. Symptoms may occur within a few weeks of first exposure but there is sometimes a latent period between removal from exposure and their onset. Prodromal symptoms such as drowsiness and vertigo are sometimes noted or alternatively, the condition may be a progression from toxic gastritis. It can also occur with no warning. The degree of jaundice is variable, but hepatic enlargement is unusual until late in the illness. Fatalities are the result of hepatic necrosis.

Aplastic anaemia is less common than toxic jaundice but invariably fatal. Like the toxic jaundice, it may occur some time after exposure has been discontinued.

Aniline: Aniline is a colourless oily liquid which turns brown on exposure to the light. It is readily absorbed through the skin and most cases of industrial poisoning are the result of accidental contamination of working clothes. Pulmonary absorption is a risk, particularly if men enter confined spaces in which the vapour is present. The closely related nitro-anilines are also absorbed through the skin. Paraphenyline diamine is considered more toxic than aniline.

Mild symptoms of intoxication take the form of flushing, a throbbing sensation in the head, burning in the throat and tightness in the chest. These are followed in turn, by the onset of a violent headache and cyanosis. It is important that exposure should cease when these early symptoms are noted. The removal of all clothing and any aniline on the skin is vital. The prognosis depends upon how much aniline has been absorbed, but in mild cases complete relief of symptoms may be expected within 24 hours. At the end of this time, the patient will no longer be cyanosed. As with the other compounds in this section, the cyanosis is due to methaemoglobinaemia. The appearance of punctate basophilia in the peripheral blood is said to be a delicate measure of increased absorption.

In severe cases of aniline poisoning, there is deep cyanosis, nausea and vomiting and circulatory collapse. The patient lapses into coma and the appearance of convulsions presages death. Characteristically, the attack occurs after the man has left work.

Chronic absorption of aniline will produce a low-grade anaemia with cyanosis which resolves when the man leaves work at the end of the day. The manifestation of symptoms will depend upon the degree of anaemia.

Aliphatic nitrates

The most important of these compounds are ethylene glycol dinitrate (EGDN) and nitroglycerin (NG) which are used to produce dynamite, a mixture of about 60 per cent ammonium and sodium nitrate, 20 per cent EGDN, 5 per cent NG, 3 per cent nitrocellulose and a variable amount of sawdust, chalk and rhodamin.

Both NG and EGDN are readily absorbed through the skin and the dust is also absorbed through the lungs. Both compounds are highly reactive and rapidly disappear from the blood. NG is metabolized to inorganic nitrates and nitrites which appear in the urine; the principal metabolites of EGDN are 1,2- and 1,3-glyceryl dinitrate.

Both NG and EGDN are potent vasodilators and the acute effects which follow exposure are the result of this property. The symptoms include throbbing hadache, tachycardia, palpitation, nausea and vomiting. Most workers become habituated to these effects so that they are noted only on return to work after 1 or 2 days absence. Sudden deaths have also been noted amongst dynamite workers. These occur typically on a Monday morning and may be preceded by symptoms which mimic those of angina pectoris. Whether dynamite workers are at risk from chronic effects is less clear. They may certainly develop hypotension at work but this appears to be a reversible phenomenon with no untoward sequelae; a few workers may also be found with a high incidence of ectopic beats on ambulatory monitoring. Epidemiological studies tend to suggest that, with present levels of exposure, the risk of death from cardiovascular disease is not substantially greater than in the general population.

PESTICIDES

Hundreds of organic compounds are used as pesticides but they can conveniently be grouped together for discussion into organochlorines, organophosphorus derivatives, carbamates and compounds related to pyrethrum.

Organochlorines

This group includes DDT, lindane (hexachlorocyclohexane), dieldrin and related chlorinated cyclodienes and hexachlorobenzene. All the organochlorine pesticides are lipid soluble and are easily absorbed by all routes. They are extremely persistent in the environment and may produce adverse effects on animals at the top of the food chain, with the general exception of man. In recent years attempts have been made to replace these compounds with others which are more readily broken down. Residues of organochlorine compounds can be measured in fat but relatively little is known about urinary metabolites.

DDT

DDT (dichloro-diphenyl trichloroethane) is an organo-chlorine compound and a most effective insecticide. It is a very stable chemical and its widespread use has resulted in a considerable accumulation in the environment which has given rise to fears that it might somehow disturb the delicate ecological balance.

The compound is absorbed through the gut and through intact skin. Once in the body, DDT undergoes a slow series of metabolic changes, the principle products of which are DDE, stored in fatty tissues and DDA, which is excreted in the urine.

In high doses, DDT affects the central nervous system, and symptoms of intoxication include paraesthesiae, tremors and convulsions. Untoward effects are not generally observed with doses less than 10 mg/kg body weight, hence cases of acute poisoning are confined to those who ingest large amounts accidentally or with suicidal intent. In fact, few fatalities have been recorded and complete recovery is the rule.

Occupational exposure is not sufficiently great to produce symptoms of acute intoxication although peripheral neuropathy has been ascribed to chronic occupational exposure. Some induction of liver enzymes can be demonstrated to have taken place in men occupationally exposed to DDT but there is no evidence of liver dysfunction of the kind which has been demonstrated in experimental animals.

Lindane

Lindane (hexachlorocyclohexane) exists in five isomeric forms. The γ-isomer is a powerful insecticide and goes under a variety of trade names of which gammexane and BHC are probably the best known. It is more toxic to insects than DDT but does not have such a long activity and on this account is sometimes used in combinatin with DDT.

Toxic effects are noted only in those who use BHC carelessly or improperly and although skin rashes have been observed in men working with BHC, these were probably due to impurities present in the compound. Individuals have poisoned themselves by taking BHC as a vermifuge, or by using the powder or a solution in poorly ventilated spaces, or by splashing their skin with the solution. Those who have been poisoned develop colic, diarrhoea, headaches, lassitude and vertigo. Neurological symptoms are prominent including ataxia, tremor and convulsions. Bone marrow depression has been recorded and some cases have ended fatally.

Users of BHC should be warned not to spray it in confined spaces, not to get it on their skin and not to take it for therapeutic purposes.

Chlorinated cyclodienes

Dieldrin is the most commonly used of the chlorinated cyclodiene pesticides. Others in this group include endrin, aldin and isodrin. Dieldrin and endrin are the most stable of the group; aldin is readily changed to dieldrin and isodrin to endrin.

All four compounds are readily absorbed through intact skin and this is the usual route of absorption for those occupationally exposed. The compounds, or their metabolites, are stored in fatty tissues but clearance from the body is accelerated by microsomal enzyme inducers such as phenobarbitone or DDT.

The most serious manifestation of acute intoxication is the production of epileptiform fits which can be well controlled with anticonvulsants. Long-term exposure to sub-toxic levels does not seem to have any untoward effects.

Hexachlorobenzene

Hexachlorobenzene is used as a fungicidal dressing for seed grain, especially wheat. It is relatively little used in Britain and no cases of occupational poisoning are known, but episodes of cutaneous porphyria have been reported from Turkey amongst villagers who have eaten seed dressed with hexachlorobenzene.

Organophosphorus compounds

These compounds are structurally related to di-iso-propyl fluoro phosphate and, like it, are powerful irreversible inhibitors of cholinesterase.

Metabolism: Organophosphorus compounds are readily absorbed through the skin as well as by ingestion and inhalation. They do not accumulate in the body and most are rapidly degraded and excreted. The principal urinary metabolites are alkyl phosphates, for example, dimethylphosphate (formed from dimethylparathion), diethylphosphate (from parathion, disulphoton and phorate), diethylphorothiolate (from disulphoton and phorate) and diethylthiophosphate (from disulphoton and phorate). In addition, p-nitrophenol is formed from parathion.

Poisoning: The toxic properties of these compounds to man lies in their ability to inhibit cholinesterase; symptoms will begin to appear when the ChE activity is reduced to less than 50 per cent of normal. Early signs of poisoning are non-specific and include headache, nausea, anorexia and marked lassitude. There may be constriction of the pupils. In a short time following exposure these relatively mild symptoms are superseded by vomiting, diarrhoea, abdominal pain and muscle twitching. Incontinence of urine and faeces is common as is pulmonary oedema. The onset of convulsions usually signifies that the patient is about to pass into a coma which may lead to his death. The complete course from exposure to death may take as little as an hour so that speed is of the essence if treatment is to be successful.

Treatment with atropine should be given immediately and the patient supported with mechanical respiration if necessary. Cholinesterase activity can be restored by compounds which split the enzyme from its attachment to the phosphate group of the insecticide. Pralidoxime is satisfactory for this purpose and a number of hospitals hold supplies of this drug for emergency purposes.

Late sequelae of organophosphorus poisoning have been noted. The patient may recover from the acute phase but about 3 weeks later note progressive muscular weakness and fatigue with vomiting and diarrhoea. Marked muscle wasting may follow. These symptoms are similar to those of TOCP poisoning *(q.v.).*

To avoid these late complications, all patients who have an attack of acute poisoning should be kept under close observation until their cholinesterase activity (in either the plasma or the red cell) has returned to normal.

Carbamates

The most important of this group is carbaryl (1-naphthyl-N-methylcarbamate) which is absorbed by all routes. It is rapidly metabolized to free and conjugate 1-naphthol which appears in the urine. The carbamates are also ChE inhibitors and produce the same kinds of symptoms as the organophosphorus insecticides. Their inhibition is rapidly reversible, however, so that they do not pose as serious a threat to health as the organophosphorus compounds.

Pyrethrum

Pyrethrum is an insecticide derived from plants. There are six active compounds, esters of two acids and three alcohols; they are known as pyrethrin I and II, cinerin I and II and jasmolin I and II. Pyrethrum may be absorbed through the gut and through the lungs but not through the skin. It is rapidly metabolized and excreted in the urine; the precise nature of its metabolites is unknown. Pyrethrum is a sensitizer and most of its untoward effects in man result from this property. Contact dermatitis is well known and it is often made worse by exposure to sunlight; signs and symptoms like those of hayfever may also be induced and there have been occasional reports of effects on the lung (see Chapter 6).

HERBICIDES

Phenoxy acid derivatives

These include 2,4-dichlorophenoxyacetic acid (2,4-D) and 2,4,5-trichlorophenoxy acetic acid (2,4,5-T) both of which have excited a great deal of alarm and despondency in recent years, particularly since 2,4,5-T has been found to be contaminated with minute traces of dioxin (2,3,7,8-tetradibenzo p-dioxin). The phenoxy acid compounds are rapidly absorbed through skin, lungs and gut and rapidly eliminated unchanged in the gut. They are remarkably non-toxic to man but fears have been raised that they are teratogenic, fears which appear to be groundless. There is some epidemiological evidence that men who are exposed to them have a higher than expected incidence of lymphomas but this is still somewhat equivocal.

Dioxin is not used commercially and is a by-product of the formation of 2,4,5-T. It is extraordinarily toxic to experimental animals but man does not share this exquisite sensitivity which is fortunate when one considers the number of industrial accidents which have resulted in environmental contamination. The most recent was at Seveso, in northern Italy. The most consistent finding in men and women exposed either at work or in the environment is chloracne and enlargement of the liver with biochemical signs of impaired liver function. There may also be an increased excretion of ALA and uroporphyrin in the urine. In man, dioxin does not seem to be notably teratogenic nor does it induce malignant disease; studies of exposed workers have been unable to demonstrate any increased prevalence of chromosomal aberrations.

Pentachlorophenol

Pentachlorophenol is used mainly as a fungicide and it can be absorbed through the skin and the gut. Fine dusts and sprays cause an intense irritation of the eyes and upper respiratory tract and provide an indication to the worker that he is over-exposing himself. The compound is excreted in the urine in free and conjugated forms.

The signs of severe intoxication include loss of appetite, respiratory distress, hyperpyrexia, sweating, anaesthesia, coma and death.

Dinitro-ortho cresol (DNOC)

This is a homologue of 4-dinitrophenol (DNP) which is also used as a fungicide and pesticide. It is absorbed by all routes and it is extremely toxic. Symptoms of poisoning are similar to those of pentachlorophenol and are likely to occur when the blood concentration is in excess of 4 mg/dl. Thirst may be an important early symptom but the most serious effects are due to interference with normal temperature regulating mechanisms; in severe cases of poisoning the patient may develop hyperpyrexia and death will supervene unless adequate treatment is quickly given.

Paraquat

Paraquat achieved a considerable notoriety at one time because of the cases of poisoning which were recorded in people who drunk the concentrated solution by accident, mistaking it for soft drinks, or with suicidal intent. Gramoxone, the 20 per cent concentrate is available only to farmers and horticulturalists and in its working strength (about 20 ppm) it is not dangerous. The form in which it is available to the public (as Weedol, a mixture of paraquat and diquat) is also harmless when used correctly. The lethal dose in man is 6 g paraquat ion (about 30 ml of gramoxone) and no one who has taken a dose in excess of this has been known to survive.

Following ingestion the patient experiences a burning sensation in the mouth and throat and has abdominal pain accompanied by nausea and vomiting. These early symptoms are followed by hepatic and renal failure, the last being due to proximal tubular damage.

The patient often survives the acute phase but after 5 to 10 days of apparently good health begins to show signs of respiratory distress. This progresses rapidly and death from respiratory failure ensues. The pathological lesion in the lungs is one of pulmonary fibrosis with an exuberant fibrotic reaction which obliterates the alveoli. The fibrotic reaction is thought to develop in response to a metabolite produced in the liver.

In order for the patient to have any chance of survival treatment must be instigated with the greatest speed. Absorption from the gut is slow and in the first 24 hours only about 10 per cent of an ingested dose is taken up; the first stage of treatment, therefore, is to perform gastric lavage using absorbents such as Fuller's earth in saline. After lavage is complete, 500 ml of a 30 per cent solution should be left in the stomach to adsorb any paraquat which remains. Haemoperfusion and haemodialysis have all been tried and treatment with steroids or immunosuppressive drugs may be given.

The prognosis in an individual case can be given on the basis of a simple examination of the urine. Paraquat is reduced to a free blue radical by alkaline sodium dithionite. If 2 ml of the reagent (freshly prepared by adding 10 ml of 1M sodium hydroxide to 100 mgm of sodium dithionite) is added to 10 ml of clear urine, the colour produced may be compared with that obtained from test solutions (containing 1, 5 and 10 mgm/l of paraquat). The test is sensitive enough to detect about 1 mgm/l of paraquat in urine. If there is no colour reaction it is safe to assume that a toxic amount of paraquat has not been ingested, whereas a colour change indicates the need for urgent treatment. Under the same test conditions, diquat is reduced to a green free radical so that a greeny-blue discoloration in the urine indicates that weedol has been ingested.

OTHER ORGANIC COMPOUNDS

Methyl bromide

Uses: Methyl bromide is an extremely volatile liquid which is in gaseous form at temperatures above 4.5°C. It is used as a fire extinguisher (sometimes mixed with carbon tetrachloride), as a refrigerant, as an insecticide and a fumigant.

Hazards of use: The danger comes from the leakage of gas from storage vessels or from faults in delivery pipes and so on. Its great volatility enables a large volume of gas to escape from even a trivial leak and its high density relative to air (it is 3.3 times as heavy as air) adds to the danger. Any process involving methyl bromide which is carried out indoors is potentially dangerous.

Metabolism: The gas is absorbed through the lungs and the skin and stored in tissues rich in fat. It is slowly broken down with the release of free bromide and measurements of the level of bromide in the blood are useful as a guide to exposure, although they do not correlate absolutely with the degree of toxicity. There are two phases of excretion; unchanged gas is excreted rapidly through the lungs, whereas bromide is excreted slowly through the kidney.

Poisoning: Methyl bromide is highly toxic but there is a latent period between exposure and the declaration of symptoms which can be as long as 48 hours. At high concentrations the gas has a slightly sweet smell.

The major effect which is noted immediately upon exposure to the gas is an irritation of the respiratory tract. Individuals thus, quickly remove themselves from further exposure. There is little narcotic action by contrast with the chlorinated hydrocarbons. After the latent interval, the patient is suddenly seized with nausea and vomiting, headaches, watering of the eyes, cough, anorexia and abdominal pain. The vision becomes blurred and the patient may have diplopia. At this stage he appears to be drunk having a staggering gait, slurred speech and vertigo. In severe cases pulmonary oedema and oliguria may occur and epilepti-form convulsions may develop.

The prognosis depends upon the length of exposure and the con-centration of the gas to which the patient was exposed. Mild forms of poisoning usually recover but it may be up to 18 months before recovery is complete. Sequelae include lassitude, peripheral neuropathy, tremor, uraemia and a variety of psychiatric symptoms such as depression, hallucinations, amnesia and insomnia.

Fatalities occur when pulmonary oedema is severe or where there is oliguria. Pathological changes in such cases include haemorrhages in the brain, liver, kidneys and lungs with small blood-stained pleural effusions. Degenerative changes are seen in the liver and kidney.

Splashes of methyl bromide on the skin produce a characteristic pattern of events. The skin is first cooled by evaporation and then a tingling, burning sensation is noted. The skin then becomes red and after several hours, small vesicles appear. The vesicles are extremely distended by straw-coloured fluid but they do not refill if they are punctured. The vesicles may coalesce. Healing takes place after a few days and is followed by a considerable desquamation.

If the degree of exposure is insufficient to produce vesicles, a dry eczematous reaction may be produced.

Treatment: No specific treatment is available and supportive measures are all that can be offered.

Tri-ortho-cresyl phosphate

Uses: Tri-ortho-cresyl phosphate (TOCP) is used in the plastics industry in great quantities as a plasticizer, i.e. a substance which renders the plastic material more pliable. It is also used in oils.

Hazards of use: The material, which is an oil with a pungent aroma, is absorbed through the skin, so all those handling it are potentially at risk. Special protective clothing, including gloves, must be worn. The oil is not very volatile and has a low vapour pressure at normal working temperatures, so inhalation is less of a risk than skin absorption. Cases of poisoning due to inhalation of the vapour have been recorded, however.

Metabolism: The compound is absorbed through the skin and becomes distributed via the blood throughout the body. The liver and spleen retain most of the absorbed material, followed by the voluntary muscles, brain and bone. Excretion takes place through the kidney.

TOCP is a potent inhibitor of pseudo-cholinesterase but has less effect on acetylcholinesterase (ChE).

Poisoning: Poisoning with TOCP develops in three stages. Initially the patient experiences mild gastro-intestinal symptoms, including nausea, vomiting, abdominal pain and diarrhoea but these subside and the patient remains well for between 1 to 3 weeks. After this interval, the distal muscles become painful and there is numbness of the fingers and toes. Bilateral foot-drop develops. There follows another interval of approximately 10 days when bilateral wrist-drop is noted. The weakness in the hands is not usually so severe as in the legs and feet, and there is no paralysis above the elbows. The signs of peripheral neuritis may be complicated by those of lower motor neurone involvement and in advanced cases the muscles of the lower limbs may be completely flaccid with absent ankle jerks. Sensory changes are not noted and loss of sphincter control is rare.

Many patients recover completely in due course but some go on to develop upper motor neurone signs with spasticity, exaggerated reflexes and marked muscle wasting. Clinically, these cases resemble those of motor neurone disease.

Cases of nonoccupational origin have been recorded due to adulteration of cooking oil with TOCP.

Resins

A vast number of resins are in industrial use as constituents of paints and varnishes, as adhesives, as sand bonders in foundry work and for making moulds. There are a great many formulations, the most common of which, arranged in order of risk, are shown in Table 4.1.

The principal risks from the use of resins are skin sensitization, with the production of an eczematous reaction, and respiratory irritation. The epoxy resins are the most active in producing skin lesions whilst the isocyanates used in polyurethane resins are the most potent producers of respiratory symptoms. The hardeners used in epoxy resins have been potent skin sensitizers and their fumes have caused asthma. Some of the constituents of other resin systems may also produce untoward effects. For example, styrene and formaldehyde used in polyester and phenolic resins respectively, both produce dermatitis and conjunctivitis and, in addition, the inhalation of formaldehyde may produce irritation of the upper respiratory tract. The conjunctivitis caused by formaldehyde may be severe and be complicated by extensive corneal damage.

ANAESTHETICS

The two anaesthetics in most common use are nitrous oxide and halothane. It goes without saying that if medical or nursing staff are overexposed in the theatre, then they will suffer the same effects, in kind if not in degree, as those of their patients. And there is good evidence that anaesthetists and other operating theatre staff suffer some behavioural effects at the end of the day. These behavioural changes are related to a depression of arousal and result, for example, in prolonged reaction times which may, in turn lead to an increased tendency to have an accident. The other effect which has been much discussed is the possibility that exposure to anaesthetic gases may cause an increased incidence of stillbirth or congenital malformation. Some American

Chapter 4

Table 4.1. Formulation of some common resin systems

System	Resins and formers	Catalyst	Curers and hardeners	Principal risks to health
High risk				
Epoxy	Epichlorhidrin aducts	Organic peroxides	Butyl glycidil ether Maleic anhydride Bisphenol polyamides	Skin sensitization
Medium risk				
Phenolic	Phenol-formaldehyde	Phosphoric acid Toluene sulphonic acid	Formaldehyde	Dermatitis, conjunctivitis and respiratory irritation from formaldehyde
Polyester	Polyesters of adipic acid and styrene monomer	Organic cobalt compounds	Organic peroxides	Dermatitis and conjunctivitis from styrene
Polyurethane	Polyesters	Amines	Isocyanates	Dermatitis and respiratory symptoms especially from TDI
Low risk				
Acrylic	Acrylic acid Acrylamide Acrylonitrile	Organic peroxides	Heat	Respiratory irritation from un-reacted acrylic compounds
Alkyd	Phthalic anhydride Glycerol		Air drying	
Furane	Furfural alcohol	Phosphoric acid Toluene sulphonic acid	Other resins	Furfural alcohol causes CNS depression

studies have showed that female operating staff have a somewhat greater relative risk for these events than other nursing or medical staff but these results have not been confirmed in the UK. Neverthless, it is prudent to minimize exposure and modern operating suites have scrubbers to remove waste gases.

Various urinary metabolites of halothane can be detected of which trifluoracetic acid is the major one. Trifluoracetic acid can also be detected in the blood and its half life is between 50–70 hours. Increased plasma bromide concentrations have also been found after exposure to halothane.

DRUGS

Some of the effects of drugs on those who manufacture or handle them are well-known. Gynaecomastia has been documented in men manufacturing synthetic oestrogens and progestogens, depression in adrenocortical function has been noted in those manufacturing steroids and sensitization has been found to a number of antibiotics. In general, however, this is not well explored territory. Some concern has recently been expressed about the hazards of handling cytotoxic drugs. The urine of nurses working on oncology wards has been found to contain mutagenic substances and also to contain a higher concentration of thioethers than nurses working in other departments. The significance of these findings to the long term health of nurses is not at all clear but there seems no reason to doubt that those who handle cytotoxic drugs will absorb a certain amount and since the drugs are mutagenic a code of practice should be followed which will minimize exposure.

CHAPTER 5/INDUSTRIAL TOXICOLOGY
4: GASES

The toxic gases may be classified into one of the three following categories:
1   Simple asphyxiants
2   Chemical asphyxiants
3   Irritants

SIMPLE ASPHYXIANTS

These gases are dangerous only when they are present in the air in a volume sufficient to diminish the partial pressure of oxygen below that which can support respiration. Nitrogen, methane and carbon dioxide are the three most important gases in this category.

Nitrogen

Nitrogen is the main constituent of chokedamp of mines, but it has industrial uses in the manufacture of ammonia and it is also used to produce an inert atmosphere for the prevention of oxidation in some metallurgical processes.

Blackdamp, which consists of about 88 per cent nitrogen and 12 per cent carbon dioxide is formed by the oxidation of the iron pyrites and calcite found in coal. It was formerly a hazard when ventilation in deep mines was inadequate and was recognized by the extinguishing of the miner's safety lamp. This occurred when the concentration of black-damp in the air was in excess of 17.7 per cent. With good ventilation in mines, blackdamp should no longer be a hazard.

Methane

Methane is known as firedamp in the mines and it became a hazard when deep shafts were first dug into the coal seams during the early part of the seventeenth century. The gas was formed in pockets in the seam and escaped when the coal was being mined. It presented two hazards to the miners, one of death from asphyxiation and one of death from the explosive mixture it formed with air. The latter danger was greatly alleviated by the introduction of the Davy Lamp in 1816, which has continued in modified form to the present day. Davy found that by interposing a metal gauze between a flame and an explosive mixture, the heat was diffused and dispersed by the gauze, so allowing the flame to burn without fear of explosion. With modern lamps the percentage of methane in the air can be estimated roughly by the height of the pale blue cap above the luminous part of the flame. In 1844 Faraday discovered that the hazard of firedamp explosion was increased by the ignition of mixtures of coal dust and air, which carried the explosion deep underground. Wet working and good ventilation have considerably reduced the hazards from firedamp.

Carbon dioxide

Carbon dioxide has a wide variety of industrial uses from the manufacture of fizzy drinks to the manufacture of freezing mixtures. It is readily liquified and is used in this form for fire extinguishers and to make carbon dioxide 'snow'. Dangerous concentrations of the gas may be encountered in mines, in fermenting vats, in breweries and mineral water factories, in coke ovens and blast furnaces and in agricultural silos and silage pits. If solid carbon dioxide is allowed to evaporate in a confined space, a dangerous concentration may build up.

Unlike the two previous asphyxiants, carbon dioxide has a powerful physiological effect and produces an increase in the respiratory rate through its action on the respiratory centre in the medulla. The symptoms produced can be related to the proportion of carbon dioxide in the atmosphere. Thus a concentration in excess of 3 per cent will produce dyspnoea which becomes pronounced when the concentration is over 5 per cent. With concentrations greater than 10 per cent, loss of consciousness supervenes after a minute or so.

The treatment of carbon dioxide poisoning consists of removing the affected person from exposure and administering oxygen.

In situations where it can be presumed that a risk from carbon dioxide might exist, the extinction of a lighted candle introduced into the oven, silo or whatever, indicates a dangerous atmosphere. Work must then only be permitted with the use of breathing apparatus. In potentially hazardous situations, men should always work in pairs.

Solid carbon dioxide can produce burns which are slow to heal. Consequently no one should be so unwise or foolhardy as to attempt to handle this substance without wearing gloves.

Chapter 5
CHEMICAL ASPHYXIANTS

Gases in this class produce their toxic effects through some sort of chemical combination with metabolically important proteins. The most important of these gases are carbon monoxide, nickel carbonyl, hydrogen sulphide, hydrogen cyanide, arsine, stibene and phosphine.

Carbon monoxide

Carbon monoxide is produced by the incomplete combustion of carbon compounds. As many of the gases used in industry contain carbon monoxide in varying proportions, there is an ever present hazard wherever they are used. The one exception is North Sea Gas which consists of methane with small amounts of butane and propane (Table 5.1). The exhaust gases of petrol and diesel engines also produce carbon monoxide and dangerous quantities may be generated in confined spaces.

Table 5.1. Chemical composition of some gases used in industry

	Carbon monoxide	Carbon dioxide	Methane	Hydrogen	Nitrogen
Coal gas	16%	2%	20%	55%	Trace
Producer gas	30%	10%	Trace	10%	50%+
Water gas	40%	5%	Trace	50%	3%
Blast furnace gas	27%	15%	Trace	2%	55%
Coke oven gas	9%	3%	25%	55%	6%
Natural gas (North Sea and Petroleum gas)	Nil	Nil	85%	Nil	Nil

In mines, carbon monoxide is the dangerous constituent of afterdamp, the gas produced during underground explosions from methane and coal dust.

Carbon monoxide is colourless and odourless and the early signs of intoxication are insidious, factors which combine to make it especially dangerous. The initial symptoms include giddiness and headache and then the patient loses the power in his legs and becomes unconscious. Concentrations of 3500 parts/10^6 are immediately hazardous to life.

Carbon monoxide has a greater affinity for haemoglobin than oxygen and combines with it to form carboxyhaemoglobin. This is a stable pigment which only slowly becomes dissociated. The symptoms of intoxication can be correlated with the carboxyhaemoglobin concentration as shown in Table 5.2. Death occurs when the blood is 60–80 per cent saturated with carboxyhaemoglobin. No cyanosis is produced, despite the profound tissue anoxia, and the patient is classically described as being cherry pink.

All those likely to be exposed to carbon monoxide should wear respirators and know how to provide first aid measures in cases of poisoning. Treatment consists of giving artificial respiration and of keeping the patient warm. The patient should be made to rest. A mixture of 95 per cent oxygen and 5 per cent carbon dioxide should be given; this is more effective in reducing the carboxyhaemoglobin saturation than oxygen alone.

Table 5.2. Correlation between carboxyhaemoglobin concentrations and symptoms of carbon monoxide poisoning

Carboxyhaemoglobin Concentration	Symptoms of Intoxication
< 20%	None except slight breathlessness on exertion.
20%–30%	Flushing, slight headache. Some breathlessness on exertion.
30%–40%	Severe headache, vertigo, nausea and vomiting, irritability and impaired judgement.
40%–50%	Symptoms as above but more severe. Fainting on exertion.
50%–60%	Loss of consciousness.
> 60%	Depression of respiratory centre leading to death.

After recovery from carbon monoxide poisoning the patient may experience severe headache. If asphyxiation has been prolonged, organic brain damage may result, with the production of lesions in the basal ganglia, dementia or depression. The elderly are more likely to be left with permanent neurological deficits than the young.

Carbon monoxide is not a cumulative poison and any gas which is absorbed during exposure to low concentrations will be excreted via the lungs when exposure has been discontinued. Many authorities dispute the existence of chronic carbon monoxide poisoning on these grounds. Nevertheless, exposure to low concentrations has been shown to impair performance in some psychological tests and in animals, to hasten the development of arteriosclerosis and produces myocardial damage.

Nickel carbonyl

Nickel carbonyl is used principally in the refining of nickel ores by the Mond process. Poisoning with this gas has two phases. Initially there is headache, nausea, vomiting and dizziness, and unconsciousness may supervene. These symptoms are very like those of carbon monoxide poisoning and in fact, carbon monoxide is always encountered with nickel carbonyl in industry.

The initial symptoms rapidly pass, to be followed in 8 to 36 hours by dyspnoea, cyanosis, weakness and pulmonary oedema. There is at first a dry cough which soon becomes worse and is accompanied by the production of blood-stained sputum. The respiratory symptoms increase in severity for about 6 days and signs of cardiac failure may be noted. Most of those affected recover with no permanent disability. In fatal cases, death occurs within 2 weeks. The final outcome depends upon the degree of damage sustained by the alveolar epithelium. At autopsy, areas of external haemorrhage are found together with atelectasis and necrosis. Haemorrhages may also be found on the brain and meninges. Supportive treatment to improve respiration is all that can be offered.

Repeated exposure to low concentrations of nickel carbonyl may give rise to a sensitivity to nickel which may in turn lead to the development of asthmatic attacks and pulmonary eosinophilia which manifests itself as patchy opacities on a chest X-ray.

Hydrogen sulphide

Hydrogen sulphide is met wherever sulphur and its compounds are worked. In mines it is called stinkdamp, for the good reason that it smells like rotting eggs. The gas is also found in gasworks, in sewers where organic matter is putrifying and in a number of chemical processes involving the manufacture of sulphur compounds.

It is at least as poisonous as hydrogen cyanide, and like HCN inhibits cytochrome oxidase by binding with ferric ions. Symptoms of intoxication will be produced when the concentration is in excess of 200 $parts/10^6$; above 600 $parts/10^6$, it is rapidly fatal.

Although the gas has such an unpleasant smell and can be detected at concentrations as low as 0.3 $parts/10^6$ above about 30 $parts/10^6$ there is a rapid accommodation to the smell which therefore increases the danger of exposure.

Once the gas is absorbed it is oxidized to a limited extent but a build-up of free hydrogen sulphide occurs. The gas can combine with methaemoglobin to form a green pigment sulphmethaemoglobin, but this does not affect tissue oxygenation.

Exposure to low concentrations causes lacrimation, photophobia, and irritation of the nasal mucosa and the pharynx. Headache, vertigo and collapse may follow. Hydrogen sulphide has a profoundly irritant effect on the cornea due to the formation of sodium sulphide, and in addition to producing pain, photophobia and lacrimation, it also causes blurring of vision and keratitis. It may cause vesicles to form on the cornea, which eventually rupture. The cornea usually recovers completely upon removal from exposure and ulceration and scarring are rare. There are no cumulative effects.

A man exposed to a high concentration of hydrogen sulphide will die immediately from the paralytic effect which the free hydrogen sulphide has on the respiratory centre in the medulla.

Treatment consists in removing the affected persons from exposure and giving oxygen. It is also worth administering amyl or sodium nitrite; the nitrite converts haemoglobin to methaemoglobin which then combines with the hydrogen sulphide to form sulphmethaemoglobin. Amyl nitrite can be given by breaking a capsule into a handkerchief which is then held over the patient's nose; sodium nitrite is given as 10 ml of a 3 per cent solution intravenously over 2 to 3 minutes, with a further 5 ml if necessary. The amount of hydrogen sulphide in work-places can be tested with lead acetate paper. At concentrations greater than 34 parts/10^6 the paper darkens immediately, at 4 parts/10^6 it will take 1 or 2 seconds to do so. Respirators should be worn by all those who are likely to be exposed to concentrations greater than 10 parts/10^6.

Hydrogen cyanide

The toxicity of this gas resides in the cyanide ion, so that all its soluble inorganic salts become hazardous under conditions which favour the release of the cyanide ion. Hydrogen cyanide in the form of potassium or sodium cyanide is used in some heat treatment or hardening processes of steel, in electroplating in the chemical industry and as a fumigant. The gas is also produced by the combustion of polyurethane foams. The poisonous properties of cyanide are well known. From time to time cyanide has enjoyed considerable popularity amongst would-be poisoners and some executioners.

Cyanide produces its action by inhibiting cytochrome oxidase thus interfering with tissue oxygenation. There is no interference with oxygen transport as is the case in carbon monoxide poisoning.

The symptoms of poisoning occur rapidly after inhalation, but if small amounts of cyanide are ingested, death may not ensue for hours. Symptoms include headache, rapid weak respirations, vomiting, excitability, tachycardia, hypotension, convulsions and coma leading to death. Pulmonary oedema and lactic acidosis may also be prominent features.

If any treatment is to be effective in a patient who is unconscious following exposure to cyanide, it must be given with all possible speed. Treatment regimes were formerly based on the production of methaemoglobin which combined with the cyanide ion to form cyanmethaemoglobin, which is nontoxic. Sodium nitrite was used intravenously to produce methaemoglobin, followed by sodium thiosulphate to convert the cyanide released by the dissociation of cyanmethaemoglobin to thiocyanate. This treatment is itself potentially hazardous and it is recommended that it be entirely superseded by treatment with di-cobalt EDTA. Six hundred mg of di-cobalt EDTA should be given intravenously and if recovery is incomplete within 1 minute, a further 300 mg is administered by the same route. Sodium thiosulphate (12.5 g in 50 ml) may be used as a supportive measure if the response to the di-cobalt EDTA is slow. During the administration of di-cobalt EDTA the patient may become hypotensive and vomiting is common. Rarely, anaphylactic reactions occur.

The symptoms of excitement and tachycardia will readily develop in anyone who supposes that he has been exposed to cyanide—understandably. However, since the poison works so rapidly, if there is an appreciable delay between presumed exposure and the development of serious symptoms, particularly drowsiness or unconsciousness, then it is most unlikely that a harmful dose has been taken. Reassurance under those circumstances may completely alleviate all symptoms.

In most cases of poisoning, the effects are so rapid that emergency treatment must be given on the spot. The man must be removed from exposure and any contaminated clothing taken off and his skin washed. Oxygen should be given if available and capsules of amyl nitrite broken into a handkerchief which is held over the patient's nose.

All personnel working in areas where cyanide is used must be instructed in its dangers and great care must be taken in the storage and handling of cyanide salts. They must not be kept where they can come into contact with acids, for example! Workers should be trained in emergency first-aid and treatment kits, containing di-cobalt EDTA must be readily available for all.

Arsine

Arsine is formed when nascent hydrogen is produced in the presence of arsenic or arsenic-containing materials. Arsenic is a contaminant of many ores including aluminium, antimony, copper, gold, lead, silver, tin and zinc, and so the formation of arsine is a hazard in the metal-working industries, especially from the action of acid on arsenic-bearing metals. The main risks are probably connected with aluminium.

The only commercial use of arsine is in the manufacture of semi-conductors in the electronics industry. The arsine is used in a carrier gas such as nitrogen in a concentration of about 100 parts/10^6. This so-called doping mixture is passed over silica crystals in a furnace where it is decomposed to form arsine which diffuses into the crystals. Excess arsine is converted to other arsenic compounds and removed by a scrubber. Other doping mixtures used in the electronics industry employ stibene, phosphine and diborane.

Arsine gradually decomposes to form pure arsenic. If cylinders of the gas are being stored or transported slight leakages of gas may result in arsenic being deposited on surfaces which could present a hazard to those handling the cylinder.

The gas is a powerful haemolytic agent and the signs and symptoms of poisoning are the result of its action on the blood. In mild cases there may be an interval of up to a day between exposure and the development of the premonitory symptoms, nausea, headache, shivering and epigastric pain. Haemoglobinuria of a high level of free haemoglobin in the plasma denote a serious degree of haemolysis. Jaundice shows on the second or third day. (It is worth noting that arsine is one of the commonest causes of toxic jaundice of occupational origin.) The jaundice is accompanied by hepatic pain and tenderness. The kidneys are severely damaged and albumin and casts are present in the urine, and anuria may be a fatal complication. The degree of anaemia clearly depends upon the extent of the haemolysis and red cell counts as low as one million/cm^3 have been recorded.

There is a considerable mortality from arsine poisoning as the result of myocardial failure. Those who survive the initial catastrophe can expect to recover fully although in some cases a peripheral neuropahy may develop which is slow to resolve. There is no specific treatment and in this respect poisoning with arsine differs from poisoning with other arsenic compounds where BAL is beneficial. Supportive measures including blood transfusion and dialysis should be given as required.

Continued exposure to very low concentrations may give rise to the development of anaemia, the true cause of which may be often un-recognized. Those who may be especially susceptible to haemolytic agents, workers with a deficiency of red cell glutathione, for example, must not be exposed at all to arsine.

Stibene

Stibene (antimony hydride) is formed accidentally when nascent hydrogen comes into contact with antimony or its compounds, when antimony alloys, or ores containing antimony are treated with acid and by wet treatment of slags or drosses contaminated with antimony.

The gas is highly toxic, colourless, but with an unpleasant smell. It rapidly decomposes at temperatures above 150°C and by contact with most oxidizing substances.

The toxic effects of stibene closely resemble those of arsine with which it may be encountered. Like arsine, it is a powerful haemolytic agent and the treatment of acute poisoning requires prompt, vigorous treatment including, when necessary, exchange transfusions and renal dialysis. There is no state of chronic poisoning.

Phosphine

Phosphine has no great commercial use and is usually met as it is evolved during manufacturing processes. It has an odour of decaying fish and is detectable in a concentration as low as 0.2 parts/10^6. At a concentration of 20 parts/10^6 it will rapidly cause death.

The gas is evolved during the preparation and use of calcium phosphide, in the manufacture of acetylene from impure calcium carbide and when zinc phosphide (sometimes used as a rat-killer) or aluminium phosphide (used to fumigate grain) are accidentally wetted. Quenching metal alloys with water may also generate the gas. Probably the main production of phosphine, however, is in the making of spheroidal graphite.

Symptoms of poisoning include abdominal pain, nausea and vomiting. Ataxia, convulsions, coma and death may supervene within 24 hours. In milder cases, the gas may produce signs of respiratory irritation and recovery is complete.

Chronic poisoning, in which neurological symptoms predominate, is said to occur in those who are continuously exposed to very low concentrations.

THE IRRITANT GASES

The irritant gases are irrespirable except at very low concentrations. Their action on the respiratory tract depends upon their solubility. Those, such as ammonia, which are readily soluble, dissolve out of the inhaled air in the upper respiratory tract and so have little effect on the lungs. Conversely, insoluble gases, such as nitrogen dioxide, penetrate the lungs and are much more injurious, causing severe pulmonary oedema.

Six gases will be considered here, ammonia, sulphur dioxide, nitrous fumes, phosgene, chlorine and fluorine.

Ammonia

Ammonia is used in great quantities in the manufacture of agricultural fertilizers. It is also used as a refrigerant, to produce an anti-oxidant atmosphere in metal furnaces and in a number of synthetic processes in the chemical industry.

The toxic effects of ammonia are due to its caustic action. If splashed on the skin it will cause a burn and enough may be absorbed to produce systemic symptoms. The vapour will cause conjunctival irritation and if splashed in the eye, conjunctivitis and keratitis will follow. More serious effects may include ulceration of the cornea and the conjunctivae which may lead to the formation of scar tissue, corneal opacities and perhaps blindness. Ammonia will rapidly penetrate the anterior chamber of the eye and it has been known to produce opacities in the lens.

Inhalation of the vapour causes a chemical bronchitis with dyspnoea, pulmonary oedema, a cough with a frothy, sometimes blood-stained sputum, tachycardia and pyrexia. In addition, ammonia vapour causes pain and oedema in the mouth and throat, with ulceration of the mucosa. Hoarseness, conjunctivitis and lacrimation are also prominent effects.

Mild cases will recover promptly on removal from exposure, although some will relapse with pulmonary oedema. Burns on the skin should be treated by copious washing with water and a buffered phosphate solution. Splashes in the eyes are treated by irrigation and corticosteroid drugs. Severe systemic effects will require hospitalization.

Men whose work involves contact with ammonia must be pre-warned of its dangers and wear gloves and goggles to prevent effects from splashing. Adequate ventilation of the work place is essential. Men who are required to repair plant where the concentration of ammonia may be high, should wear respirators.

Sulphur dioxide

Sulphur dioxide is produced by the combustion of sulphur compounds. It is used in the production of sulphuric acid, as a preservative of food and wine, as a fumigant and it was used in the past as a refrigerant. More commonly, however, it is encountered as a contaminant, both inside and outside industry. In industry it is an important contaminant in magnesium foundries, whilst in the general environment it is a notable constituent of fog and smog.

The gas has a characteristically pungent smell which can be detected when the concentration is about 3 parts/10^6. It is highly irritant to the mucous membranes of the eye and the respiratory tract. In low concentrations the vapour produces lacrimation, sneezing and coughing. Serious poisoning is rare because the gas is so irritant that those exposed rapidly run away. When escape is difficult, the patient will develop severe respiratory distress, collapse and die. Men continuously exposed to low concentrations will develop some tolerance to its effects and be able to work in a concentration containing up to 10 parts/10^6, whereas those who are unacclimatized develop symptoms when the concentration is of the order of 3 parts/10^6. Mild cases will recover with no treatment beyond removal from exposure, and the conjunctivitis heals with no sequelae. Serious cases of poisoning require treatment in hospital.

Continuous exposure to low concentrations tends to produce upper respiratory disease and partial loss of taste and smell. Abrupt increases in the concentration of sulphur dioxide to levels greater than 0.25 parts/10^6 in the atmosphere of cities is associated with a slight increase in general mortality, if at the same time smoke concentrations are also increased. Levels of sulphur dioxide greater than 0.5 parts/10^6 are associated with a 20 per cent increase in mortality compared with 'normal' mortality, but only if smoke levels are greater than 200 μg/m^3. Those who suffer most are patients with chronic pulmonary disease.

Liquid sulphur dioxide

This was widely used as a refrigerant and severe injuries to the eyes have been caused as the result of accidental splashing. The corneal epithelium swells and is shed after a few days to reveal infiltration of the stroma and interstitial vascularization. Corneal scarring, overgrowth of the cornea by conjunctival epithelium and permanent defects of vision are all late results. Prolonged irrigation of the eye with water must be undertaken as quickly as possible after liquid sulphur dioxide has gone into the eye.

Nitrous fumes

Nitrous fumes are an equilibrium mixture of the two dioxides of nitrogen, nitogen oxide (NO_2) and dinitrogen textroxide (N_2O_4) in the ratio of approximately 3 : 7; the equilibrium between the two, however, is temperature dependent. The other oxides of nitrogen are nontoxic and nitrous oxide (N_2O) is used as an anaesthetic; despite some fears to the contrary, there is no evidence that it has any neuropsychological effects at low concentrations. Nitrous fumes take the form of reddish-brown fumes, slightly heavier than air and they are produced whenever nitric acid is exposed to the air or whenever it reacts with organic material. They are also produced during the combustion of material such as celluloid, which contains a nitrous radical, by the combination of nitrogen and oxygen during such processes as oxyacetylene, carbon-arc or electric-arc welding and in mining when dynamite is used for blasting and burns quietly instead of exploding. During the fermentation of silage the fumes may also be given off as the result of the reduction of nitrogen, and men at work in silos may be affected by the fumes and get what is known as silo-fillers' disease.

Of all the irritant gases, nitrous fumes are the most insidious and since the margin between concentrations which will provoke mild symptoms and those which will produce fatal results is small, the gas is a serious danger. Moreover, workers may inhale potentially lethal amounts without the ill effects being noted for anything from 2 to 24 hours. Fortunately, workers are easily trained to take great care when they see the distinctive coloured fumes and thus avoid any ill effects.

There are three more or less distinct syndromes of poisoning with nitrous fumes. Exposure to concentrations in the range of 100–500 ppm may cause sudden bronchospasm and death from respiratory failure. The most typical consequence of exposure, however, is the development of a chemical alveolitis with severe pulmonary oedema. Upper respiratory irritation is generally mild. As a rule, the immediate symptoms which follow exposure are so mild as to escape notice, but some irritation of the eyes and throat may be noted together with a cough and some tightness in the chest. As the pulmonary oedema develops the patient will become dsypnoeic and develop a cough with much blood stained sputum. In severe cases, cyanosis, circulatory failure and death may follow. Treatment of these cases is as for any other cause of severe pulmonary oedema and complete recovery should be expected.

The third syndrome of poisoning with nitrous fumes is associated with an inflammatory response in the lungs thought to be due to an auto-immune reaction. The condition is sometimes referred to as bronchiolitis fibrosa obliterans. It is not clear whether this condition is a late sequel of acute intoxication or whether it is caused by repeated exposure to concentrations in the range 20–50 ppm.

The hazards of nitrous fumes must be made known to all who work where they are liable to be generated and measures must be taken to prevent the escape of the fumes into the general working environment. Welding processes must be carried out with adequate ventilation and oxygen must not be used to sweeten the air in confined spaces where welding is in operation. It is important to warn workers of the dangers of putting sawdust or wood shavings or any other organic material onto spilt nitric acid: it should be hosed away with large quantities of water by men wearing suitable respirators.

Chlorine

Chlorine is used for the manufacture of chlorine compounds, for bleaching paper and man-made fibres and as a disinfectant for water supplies, swimming pools and sewage. It has the doubtful distinction of being the first war gas.

The gas has a pungent, irritating odour and this usually causes those exposed to take prompt evasive action. Immediate symptoms of intoxication are choking, a retrosternal burning pain, coughing, irritation of the eyes and mouth, and excessive salivation and lacrimation. An intense headache and severe epigastric pain are common. Nausea and vomiting may follow. The patient appears acutely ill and becomes cyanosed. He may develop pulmonary oedema if the concentration of gas is high (greater than 40 parts/10^6).

Complete rest with supportive treatment is essential and can best be given in hospital. Respiratory distress can persist for up to 2 weeks but recovery is complete.

A high standard of safety is called for in those industries using chlorine and respirators must be worn for hazardous jobs. Adequate ventilation in the general working area is essential.

It is perhaps worth remembering also that chlorine may be liberated from domestic hypochlorite bleaches if they are reacted with ammonia, acids or sodium bisulphate, as may occur when bleaches of different composition are mixed.

Phosgene

Phosgene (carbonyl chloride) is used in the synthesis of several organic compounds and as an agent for direct chlorination. It may also be liberated when halogenated hydrocarbons are heated, so that welding and smoking should not be allowed where de-greasing agents such as trichlorethylene or carbon tetrachloride are in use. For the same reason, portable fire extinguishers which contain carbon tetrachloride should not be provided for use in enclosed spaces since there is a risk that the carbon tetrachloride will decompose on contact with hot metal. The use of phosgene as a war gas provided the opportunity to study the toxic effects on a wide scale: 80 per cent or more of the fatalities due to gas in the 1914–18 war were caused by phosgene.

The gas has a sweet smell, said to resemble that of green corn or geraniums. It is much more toxic than chlorine. There are no immediate symptoms following exposure to low concentrations beyond a slight irritation of the eyes and upper respiratory tract. After 24–48 hours, however, severe pulmonary oedema may develop, with circulatory collapse.

After exposure to high concentrations, the patient will notice tightness in the chest, with nausea and vomiting a few minutes after he has begun to inhale the gas. Upper respiratory tract irritation is noted and conjunctivitis develops. Pulmonary oedema with cough, cyanosis and collapse all follow suit. Any activity enhances the symptoms so complete rest is mandatory. Treatment is only practicable in hospital, bearing in mind that acute pulmonary oedema may develop after an interval as late as 48 hours.

Chest X-rays show the presence of multiple, ill-rounded shadows, and the area of the opacities correlates reasonably well with the degree of exposure.

Recovery is slow and effort syndrome is a common sequel to an attack of gassing. Repeated acute episodes can lead to chronic pulmonary disease.

Fluorine and compounds of fluorine

Fluorine is one of the most chemically active elements known. In the free state it is a green-yellow gas with a pungent smell which can be detected at low concentrations. Compounds of fluorine including fluor-spar (calcium fluoride) and cryolite (sodium aluminium fluoride) are used as fluxes in the metal industry and they are also used in the chemical industry. Clays containing calcium fluoride are used in the pottery industry and when these clays are fired, fluorosilicates are produced. These substances constitute a serious hazard. Uranium hexafluoride is used to separate uranium isotopes, whilst hydrofluoric acid is used in the manufacture of aluminium fluoride. It is also used to etch glass and in the pottery industry, to etch china prior to gold decoration. Organic fluorine compounds such as dichlorodifluoro-methane (freon) are used in refrigeration and in vast amounts as propellants in aerosol cans. Teflon, widely used as a nonstick lining for pans, is polytetrafluoroethylene.

Hydrofluoric acid

In addition to its industrial uses, hydrofluoric acid is evolved in the manufacture of super-phosphates by treating bones with sulphuric acid.

Anhydrous hydrofluoric acid is a colourless liquid, which gives off an irritant vapour. Fluorine gas is invariably converted to hydrofluoric acid by combining with the water in the atmosphere or on wet mucosal surfaces.

On the skin hydrofluoric acid produces an effect which varies from mild erythema to a severe burn, depending on the concentration and length of exposure. The burn is characterized by an intense throbbing pain which may be delayed several hours. A tough white coagulum forms over the area of damage, under which progressive destruction of all tissues continues. Burns under the finger-nails are notable in this respect because of the difficulties of treatment.

If the vapour is inhaled the larynx and the trachea are affected; there is severe retrosternal pain and cough, with sputum and perhaps hae-moptysis. Pulmonary oedema may also result. Should the liquid be swallowed, the mouth and pharynx are burned and there is nausea, vomiting and collapse. Slow ulceration of all sites in contact with the liquid or vapour is the ultimate result.

Treatment: The burns must be given immediate first aid. Contaminated clothing is removed and the area washed with copious amounts of water for 1 minute. A gel containing 2.5 per cent calcium gluconate should be applied and massaged into the burnt area and this should be continued until 15 minutes after the pain in the burn is relieved or until the patient is removed to hospital. If the area of the burn is large (greater than 65 cm^2) calcium should be given by mouth. A dose of 6 effervescent calcium tablets in water should be given every 2 hours until the patient is in hospital.

Great care must be taken by all those handling hydrofluoric acid. The liquid attacks glass and so is transported and stored in tarred barrels or metal containers. Workers must wear protective clothing and be taught to examine their gloves regularly for small holes. Face masks must be worn and good exhaust ventilation is required. Running water must be available in areas where hydrofluoric acid is handled for drenching the skin in case of burns. All workers should be instructed in the dangers of hydrofluoric acid and in how to give first aid.

Fluorosis

The chronic absorption of relatively high concentrations of fluoride ion can produce pathological changes which are largely confined to skeletal tissues. Such changes have been found in workers handling fluorspar, fluorapatite and cryolite. In addition, the condition has been found in some members of the general public living near foundries using iron ore and coal containing fluoride, and near factories manufacturing aluminium. Fluorosis has also been reported to occur in animals grazing near factories which emit fluoride, aluminium factories for example, and fertilizer and brick and ceramics factories.

The skeletal changes include the coarsening of the spongy trabeculae, periosteal new bone deposition with the formation of osteophytes, and ossification of ligaments and tendons. Bone which is severely affected is chalky-white and easily cut with a knife. Symptoms are not apparent in the early stages of the disease, but gradually vague pains are noted in the small joints of the hands and the feet. As the changes progress the patient may develop kyphosis together with limitation of spinal movement and flexion contractions of the hips and knees. Ultimately, compression of the nerve roots and spinal cord may cause the development of paraesthesiae, weakness and paralysis.

The teeth become mottled even when the intake of fluoride is relatively low, and in some parts of the world, the condition is almost unavoidable because of the high concentration of fluoride in the drinking water. Tooth mottling is a very sensitive index of chronic fluorine poisoning. The teeth show chalky-white streaks and blotches and are dotted with irregular defects in the enamel which is discoloured a light brown or black. All the permanent teeth are affected and changes in the deciduous teeth have also been recorded. Children born to some female cryolite workers have developed dental mottling as the result of absorbing fluoride excreted in their mother's milk.

Fluorides are avid bone seekers and they produce their effects by depressing collagen formation and bone resorption and by increasing bone crystal formation. There is some evidence that a high dietary intake of calcium will reduce the toxicity of ingested fluoride compounds, presumably through the formation of the relatively insoluble calcium fluoride.

At low level, fluoride in drinking water ($<$ 1 mg/litre) is said actually to be of benefit in dental hygiene, reducing the rate of decay and the incidence of caried teeth. A number of local authorities have introduced schemes for the fluoridation of public water supplies, but clearly such schemes must be rigidly controlled to prevent concentrations in excess of 1 mg/litre being presented to the general public.

Treatment: There is no specific treatment and so there is a great need to protect workers from absorbing the dust generated during smelting of fluoride ores. Such processes should be exhaust ventilated and as much of the handling as possible carried out mechanically. Masks should be worn by those likely to be in contact with the dust.

Polytetrafluorethylene

Polytetrafluorethylene (PTFE) begins to decompose when heated to temperatures of about 250°C, producing hydrogen fluoride and a range of aliphatic and cyclic saturated and unsaturated compounds. At higher temperatures, sulphur dioxide, carbon monoxide, chlorine, phosgene and perfluoroisobutylene may all be evolved, the last being extremely toxic.

Inhalation of these breakdown products produces an illness known as polymer fume fever which resembles metal fume fever. Smoking cigarettes contaminated with PTFE is the most common cause of the illness, the cigarettes becoming contaminated either from the workers' hands or from specks of PTFE powder which settle onto the lighted end of the cigarettes from the air.

The symptoms of the illness include fever and shivering, and a cough with tightness in the chest. In rare cases pulmonary oedema has been recorded.

The symptoms subside within 24 to 48 hours and there are no sequelae. No syndrome of chronic poisoning is known.

CHAPTER 6/OCCUPATIONAL
LUNG DISEASE

OBSTRUCTIVE AIRWAYS DISEASE

Occupational asthma

Occupational asthma is a disease characterized by reversible airways obstruction which is causally related to exposure of a variety of agents in the workplace. It is a disease which is becoming increasingly prevalent. There are in excess of 200 agents which have been reported to cause occupational asthma; the most important are shown in Table 6.1. In some cases (shown in the Table), sufferers from occupational asthma are entitled to compensation. The prevalence of occupational asthma amongst groups at risk is not known with certainty but such studies as have been carried out suggest that it may be high. For example, up to a third of new entrants to platinum refining leave within 18 months because they develop asthma and a similar proportion of those using colophony resin in the electronics industry may be affected. Between 5–10 per cent of those handling laboratory animals may develop asthma and be forced to find other work and up to half of those who handle locusts are affected; this might be a case of the animals fighting back.

There is always a variable interval between first exposure and the development of symptoms which may vary from a few weeks to several years. The symptoms of an attack may develop within minutes of exposure (the immediate type) or some hours after first exposure, perhaps long after the patient has left work (non-immediate type). In the immediate type of attack the symptoms tend to be maximal within 10 to 20 minutes of onset and last for up to 2 hours. In the non-immediate type, the symptoms are maximal within 4 to 8 hours and often recover within 24 hours. It should not be thought that the differentiation is always clear cut, however, and intermediate types occur. Nor does the occurrence of immediate symptoms exclude the possibility of late symptoms for, in some unfortunate individuals, both occur. In some cases there is a tendency for symptoms to recur at about the same time on a number of successive nights following a single exposure. This is sometimes referred to as late recurrent asthma or recurrent nocturnal asthma.

Table 6.1. Main agents known to cause occupational asthma

Biological agents
Enzymes of *B. subtilis* (e.g. alcalase)*
Colophony resin (used as soft solder flux)*
Urinary proteins of small mammals (e.g. rats, mice, guinea pigs)*
Grains and flours and their contaminants (e.g. moulds, mites)*
Wood dusts (e.g. Western red cedar, Iroko)
Drugs (e.g. penicillin, cephalosporins)
Insects (e.g. locusts, cockroaches, stick insects)

Chemical agents
Di-isocyanates including toluene (TDI), diphylmethane (MDI), hexamethylene
  (HDI), and naphthalene (NDI)*
Complex salts of platinum (especially ammonium hexaplatinate)*
Acid anhydride hardening agents including epoxy resin curing agents (e.g. phthalic,
  trimellitic acid and tetrachlorophthallic acid anhydrides)*
Formaldehyde

---

*Causes for which compensation is awarded in the UK.

The diagnosis of occupational asthma depends to a large degree on the examining physician bearing the possibility in mind. It should always be considered when asthma first comes on in adult life. Wheeze is not always the most prominent symptom and in many cases all the patient will complain of is a cough or a little breathlessness. Those who are affected, however, will often appreciate that their symptoms develop at work and may increase in severity as work progresses; the cardinal feature to elicit from the history is that—in the early stages at least—the symptoms improve away from work, over the weekend or on holiday.

A history of atopy is not always helpful in making the diagnosis since, although there is an increased risk for atopic subjects to develop asthma when exposed to some sensitizers (grain dust, platinum salts, detergents and locusts, for example), many of those who develop occupational asthma are non-atopic. Because the results of skin prick tests may be negative, many cases of occupational asthma are diagnosed as having intrinsic asthma; others who smoke may be mistakenly said to have chronic bronchitis, especially if a productive cough is prominent amongst the symptoms.

The most helpful aid to diagnosis is self-measurement of the peak expiratory flow rate (PEFR) at 2 hour intervals throughout the day using a simple peak flow meter. Routine measurement of lung function before and after a working shift is often exceedingly unhelpful and may be downright misleading. The patient is asked to read his PEFR for several days including a week-end and preferably a longer period away from work. Two weeks is generally the minimum for which readings should be taken. The patient must be carefully instructed in the test procedure and he must continue with his normal work whilst taking measurements and a note should be made of any bronchodilators which are taken, and their dose should not be varied throughout the period of observation. Drugs which would block the changes in the airways in response to sensitizers (corticosteroids or sodium cromoglycate) should be withheld.

In non-asthmatics the diurnal variation in PEFR will generally be less than 10 per cent whereas in asthmatics it is usually greater than 20 per cent. Depending on the time taken for lung function to recover, four patterns maybe seen in PEFR records.

1   There may be progressive deterioration throughout the working week in which case the reduction in lung function is greater at the end than the beginning of the week and recovery may take up to 3 days. If recovery takes only 1 or 2 days and is substantial, then the weekly pattern is regular. If it takes the full 3 days and a late reaction occurs on the first day at work, the lung function on that day is the best of the week and it maybe reduced throughout the weekend.

2   If deterioration is more or less the same on each day and recovery after leaving work is rapid, then the pattern will be the same on each working day and normal on the days away from exposure.

3   If recovery takes longer than 3 days then there will be a progressive decline week by week until a fixed state is reached. Following cessation of exposure recovery may not begin for a week or two and not be complete for as long as 3 months.

4   Rarely in occupational asthma, the deterioration in PEFR may be most pronounced on the first day of exposure and may recover throughout the rest of the week. This type of response is typical of humidifier fever and byssinosis.

Skin prick tests can be elicited in sensitive individuals by a number of soluble allergens including those in wheat and rye flour and rat and mouse urine, alcalase and ammonium hexachloroplatinate. An immediate wheal and flare reaction indicates the presence of a specific IgE antibody to the allergen and provides corroborative evidence for the diagnosis; a negative reaction does not exclude it.

Testing for specific antibodies in serum is not as yet of great help in making a diagnosis although IgE and IgG antibodies have been found against TDI, MDI, trimellitic and phthallic anhydrides and ammonium hexachloroplatinate.

In a number of well defined circumstances it may be necessary to undertake inhalation bronchial provocation tests; these must be carried out in hospital by a physician experienced in their use. The indications for provocation tests are if the patient's symptoms are so severe that it would be hazardous to allow him to return to work to carry out peak flow measurements; if the putative allergen is not one already recognized as causing occupational asthma; if the patient is exposed to more than one agent at work or if a diagnosis cannot be reached by any other means.

Management and prognosis

If exposure can be entirely discontinued the prognosis is good although in some cases the symptoms may be prolonged and disabling; in these cases there may be cross-reactivity with other allergens. Very often the only way in which exposure can be totally avoided is if the individual is relocated within his place of work of if he finds another job. Neither may be easy and the individual may prefer to stay where he is. If this is his choice, then he must be offered some form of personal protection which will reduce exposure to the bare minimum—air flow helmets have often been found effective—and he may require prophylactic medication. Atopics should be excluded only from occupations which involve exposure to platinum salts, *B. subtilis* enzymes and grain and flour dusts; they ought also to avoid locusts.

Pathogenic mechanisms

Early asthmatic responses are caused by the interaction of antigen with IgE antibodies with subsequent release of histamine and other bronchoactive substances from the mast cell; in some cases short-term sensitizing IgG antibodies may also be involved. Early symptoms are prevented by pre-treatment with sodium cromoglycate.

The mechanism by which the non-immediate symptoms are produced is less clear but it is probable that in most cases IgE is the specific antibody since they also may be prevented by sodium cromoglycate which inhibits the release of histamine from the mast cell.

Byssinosis

Byssinosis is a disease peculiar to textile workers. It begins with tightness in the chest and breathlessness after a long period of exposure to cotton, flax, hemp or sisal dusts, commonly of the order of several years.

Table 6.2. Clinical grades of byssinonis

Grade	Symptoms
C½	Occasional tightness of the chest on the first day of the working week.
C1	Tightness of the chest and/or difficulty in breathing on each first day only of the working week.
C2	Tightness of the chest and/or difficulty in breathing on the first and other days of the working week.
C3	Grade C2 symptoms accompanied by evidence of permanent respiratory disability from reduced ventilatory capacity.

There is some evidence that byssinosis is more common in atopics than non-atopics and it is distinct from the other diseases which may follow exposure to these dusts, mill fever, weavers' cough and mattress makers' fever (qv). The symptoms of byssinosis can be classified into four clinical grades (Table 6.2). Those of grades C½ to C2 behave like those of a late asthma, that is, there is a delay of some hours between the start of exposure and their onset, but the disease can be differentiated from asthma on the grounds that it recovers during the week. The symptoms of grade C3 appear to represent irreversible airways obstruction and the association with smoking is so great that it is difficult to be certain that this grade is an entity which is truly distinct from chronic bronchitis. Recovery from grades C½ to C1 will be complete if exposure is discontinued but slight impairment will probably remain in individuals in C2. Individuals in C3 may go on to develop right heart failure. The asthmatic symptoms are relieved by bronco-dilators and antihistamines and are probably caused by histamine liberators in the dusts; the extent to which there is also an immunological aetiology is uncertain.

The symptoms first appear on a Monday, usually several hours after the start of exposure, and the man may be well for the rest of the week. As the disease progresses the symptoms extend further into the week until a state of permanent breathlessness with cough and sputum becomes established. There is no fibrotic change in the lungs and chest X-rays show no distinguishing features although individuals in C3 may have emphysematous changes.

Changes in lung function

The magnitude of the effect on the dust exposure can be determined by measuring the FEV_1 at the start and the end of the shift. For epidemiological purposes the differences between these values can be graded as follows:

F0: No demonstrable acute effect and no evidence of chronic ventilatory impairment;

F½: Slight acute effect; no chronic impairment;

F1: Moderate acute effect;

F2: Evidence of slight to moderate irreversible impairment, and

F3: Moderate to severe irreversible impairment.

Mill fever

This is a mild febrile condition which occurs only on first contact with cotton, flax, hemp or kapok dust. The fever is accompanied by a slight cough and rhinitis. The symptoms are mild and disappear as exposure continues. They are probably caused by endotoxins derived from Gram-negative bacteria in the dusts. It has been suggested that byssinosis does not occur in individuals who have no previous history of mill fever.

Weavers' cough

This was a form of late asthma accompanied by fever and malaise. The symptoms occurred in those handling cotton yarns treated with flour paste or tamarind seed extract and were thought to be caused by contaminating fungi.

Mattress maker's fever

This was probably a form of extrinsic allergic alveolitis occurring in workers handling cotton contaminated by *Aerobacter cloacae.* The symptoms began within 6 hours of exposure and consisted of fever, malaise, nausea and vomiting; asthma did not occur.

GRANULOMATA

Foreign body granulomata may be found in association with talc pneumoconiosis (see below) whilst granulomata resembling those seen in sarcoid are a prominent feature of the acute phase of extrinsic allergic alveolitis and the chronic stage of beryllium poisoning.

Extrinsic allergic alveolitis

This condition is the classic example of a Type III mediated hyper-sensitivity reaction. The antigen is typically a fungal protein and some of the causes are shown in Table 6.3.

Of the conditions listed in Table 6.3 those most frequently en-countered are farmer's lung and bird fancier's lung. The former results from the inhalation of spores of *Microspora faeni* and *Thermoactinomyces vulgaris* growing in mouldy hay. The latter is caused by the inhalation of dried serum proteins contained in the faeces of birds. Owners of pigeons and budgerigars are those most often affected.

Table 6.3. Some causes of occupation extrinsic allergic alveolitis

Condition	Origin of dust	Causative agent
Farmer's lung	Mouldy hay	*Micropolyspora faenia* and *Thermoactinomyces vulgaris*
Bird fanciers' lung	Bird droppings and feathers	Avian proteins
Bagassosis	Mouldy sugar cane	*T. sacchari*
Mushroom pickers' lung	Mushroom compost	*M. faeni* and *T. vulgaris*
Malt workers' lung	Mouldy malt and barley	*Aspergillus clavatus* and *A. fumigatus*
Wheat weevil lung	Grain and flour dust infected with wheat weevil	*Sitophilus granarius*
Maple bark disease	Mouldy maple bark	*Cryptostroma corticale*
Animal handlers' lung	Dust of dander, hair particles and dried urine	Serum and urinary proteins
Cheese washers' lung	Mould dust	*Penicillium casei*
Fish meal workers' lung	Fish meal dust	Fish proteins
Di-isocyanate alveolitis	TDI and HDI vapour and dust	TDI and HDI
Suberosis	Mouldy cork dust	*P. frequentans*
Pyrethrum alveolitis	Insecticide aerosol	Pyrethrum
Paprika splitters' lung	Mouldy red peppers	*Mucor stolinifer*

Bagassosis is a disease of men inhaling the fibrous residue of sugar-cane stalks after the juice has been extracted by crushing. This bagasse is used for a number of purposes, including the manufacture of fibre boards. The hazard arises when the bagasse is dry and mouldy.

Malt workers' lung occurs in distilling and brewery workers handling fungally contaminated grain whilst cheese makers' lung is observed in those engaged in washing moulds off Swiss cheese. Grain workers, animal handlers and those exposed to di-isocyantes may, in addition to asthma, also show the signs and symptoms of allergic alveolitis with basal crepitations and impairment of gas transfer. Fish meal workers' lung was observed in a factory manufacturing animal food in which fish meal was incorporated but allergic alveolitis following exposure to pyrethrum-based insecticides has only been observed following over-exposure in the home. Maple-bark stripper's lung occurs in men working in paper mills and has been controlled by spraying the logs during de-barking and by issuing respirators to those at risk. Mushroom workers' lung is an uncommon variety of extrinsic allergic alveolitis and of the remaining types shown in Table 6.3, paprika splitters' lung and suberosis do not occur in this country. Indeed the former is now an historical curiosity. It used to be found amongst the Hungarian women who picked and processed a certain variety of red peppers, but the paprika splitter has been made redundant by advances in horticulture which have produced peppers which need no human processing and with their disappearance has gone the disease. Suberosis is a problem amongst the cork workers in Portugal and arises from the inhalation of mouldy cork dust. Clean cork dust does not cause pulmonary disease.

The symptoms of the disorder are the same irrespective of the external agent although they may vary in severity. After an interval of 4 to 6 hours, an influenza-like illness develops during which the patient feels unwell, has pains in the limbs and is febrile. The patient also has a dry cough and dyspnoea but no wheeze. The only abnormal sign in the chest is the presence of scattered crepitations heard throughout the lung field. After 2 to 3 days the symptoms abate.

Repeated acute attacks of extrinsic allergic alveolitis may lead to the development of chronic changes in the lungs. These give rise to progressive respiratory failure and sometimes to airways obstruction. Evidence of cor pulmonale may be found. A few patients have finger clubbing with persistent crepitations.

In acute attacks the chest X-rays show changes which vary from a diffuse haze to widespread nodular shadowing. Chronic changes include shadowing, often most predominant in the upper zones, and honey-combing.

Pathologically the typical feature of the acute phase is the presence of granulomata in the walls of the alveoli and respiratory bronchioles. The granulomata contain multinuclear giant cells and lymphocytes, and plasma cells are common. In chronic cases the normal lung architecture is destroyed producing fibrosis and honey-combing.

In farmers' lung the presence of circulating antibodies is found in asymptomatic farmers as well as in those with symptoms and thus has no diagnostic value. The demonstration of antibodies to pigeon proteins is also of no great diagnostic value since about 40 per cent of symptomless pigeon owners have antibodies. By contrast, the presence of antibodies to budgerigar serum almost always reflects clinical disease. Considerably cross-reactivity occurs from one avian species to another so that an individual sensitive to one bird may develop symptoms when exposed to another species with which he does not normally come into contact.

Patients with bird-fanciers' lung have an increased frequency of HLA-B8 antigens, which is interesting in the context of the changes found in the gut since this is also the case with patients who have coeliac disease, and it is tempting to postulate a common aetiological link. However, HLA-B8 is also more common in patients with farmers' lung, in whom gut symptoms have not been noted, so the significance of this observation is not yet clear.

Thesaurosis

Granulomata may develop in the lung following the inhalation of natural or synthetic resins. Thesaurosis is the name given to a sarcoid-like illness which has been reported in a small number of hairdressers and alleged to be due to the inhalation of hair lacquer spray. The patients had complaints of breathlessness and showed radiological changes characteristic of early sarcoid with hilar lymphadenopathy and widespread miliary infiltrates. When exposure to the hair spray was discontinued, the patients made a spontaneous recovery.

Vine-yard sprayers' lung

This is a disease found amongst those who are engaged in spraying the French vineyards with Bordeaux solution which contains dilute copper sulphate. After a number of years of exposure, the affected workers develop dyspnoea and their chest X-rays show the presence of nodular and linear shadows. The nodules are granulomata which contain copper.

Humidifier fever

This is a condition which has some of the features of alveolitis, whilst being accompanied by constitutional symptoms like those of metal fume fever. The characteristic feature of all the case reports is that the patients have been inhaling air contaminated by micro-organisms which have been dispersed from humidifiers of various sorts.

The major complaints are those of malaise, fever, cough, tightness in the chest and myalgia which develop within a few hours of starting work and which usually improve within 24 hours. These symptoms are worse on Monday mornings and may be accompanied by breathlessness and a cough. There are no radiological abnormalities, but physiological studies show impaired gas transfer and reduction in ventilatory capacity.

The micro-organisms responsible for the symptoms grow in the water which is recirculated through the humidifying system and from it, bacteria, protozoa and fungi of many kinds have been cultured. Most of those affected have serum precipitins to the crude water extract and the symptoms can generally be reproduced when the victims cautiously inhale extracts of the contaminated water. The immunological basis of the disease has not yet been worked out and it has been shown that workers without symptoms may also have precipitins in their serum.

The disease can be abolished by using steam humidifiers instead of those which depend upon re-circulating water and steam humidifiers are recommended for all new installations.

A similar disease has been described in workers in sewage disposal plants in which sludge is thermally reduced to powder. It is thought that the symptoms are a response to the protein from the high concentration of Gram negative bacteria in the environment.

Legionnaires' disease

This is an atypical pneumonia caused by *Legionella pneumophila* of which there are over 20 species with 10 serogroups. The disease is not strictly occupational but since the causative organism is ubiquitous in water it has occurred in those working in large buildings with infected water systems including hotels and hospitals. The disease has no distinguishing clinical or radiological features and diagnosis is based on finding specific antibodies using an indirect fluorescent antibody test. It can be treated effectively with erythromycin or rifampicin and prevented by chlorinating the water to a concentration of 2–4 ppm or by heating it to between 55–60°C.

Beryllium disease

Chronic beryllium disease is the other granulomatous disease of major occupational significance and is discussed in Chapter 2.

CHEMICAL PNEUMONITIS

Chemical pneumonitis with pulmonary oedema follows the inhalation of many toxic gases and fumes because of damage to the respiratory epithelium and the alveolar capillaries. The more important are the halogens, nitrous fumes, sulphur dioxide, phosgene and the fumes of cadmium. Further details are to be found in Chapters 2 and 5.

PNEUMOCONIOSIS

The term pneumoconiosis is used as a generic name to cover the group of lung disorders which result from the inhalation of dust. Many of these dusts give rise to a fibrotic reaction in the lung with the production of overt clinical symptoms, but there is also a group of dusts of high radio-density which cause opacities on chest X-rays but no symptoms. These radiographic changes are sometimes referred to as those of benign penumoconiosis. The opacities are due to the fact that the inhaled dusts contain minerals whose atomic number is high enough to cause significant X-ray absorption. The density of the opacities produced by these dusts is directly proportional to their atomic number.

Table 6.4. Outline of the short ILO classification of the radiographic changes seen in pneumoconiosis

Feature	Classification
No pneumoconiosis	0
Pneumoconiosis	
SMALL OPACITIES	
Rounded	
Profusion	1, 2, 3
Type	p, q(m), r(n)
Extent	—
Irregular	
Profusion	1, 2, 3
Type	s, t, u,
Extent	—
LARGE OPACITIES	
Size	A, B, C
Type	—

The International Labour Office (ILO) has issued a standard method for the classification of the radiographic changes seen in pneumoconiosis and an outline of the short classification is shown in Table 6.4. The object of the classification is to enable the radiographic changes seen in penumoconiosis to be coded in a simple reproducible form. It does not define pathological entities nor enable any assessment to be made of working capacity.

The classification has found world-wide acceptance and it is used in this country by the Pneumoconiosis Medical Panels.

The benign pneumoconioses

These are only recognized during life by the presence of small, rounded, dense opacities (ILO categories p or q) on a chest film which are caused by perivascular collections of dust.

Siderosis (iron-oxide lung) is the most common of the benign

Explanation of symbols in Table 6.4

Small opacities

Rounded	Irregular
Type	
p = up to 1.5 mm diameter	s = fine, irregular or linear opacities
*q(m) = > 1.5 mm but < 3 mm diameter	t = medium opacities
*r(n) = > 3 mm but < 10 mm diameter	u = coarse opacities

Profusion

0 = opacities absent or less profuse than in Category 1.	0 = opacities absent or less profuse than in Category 1.
1 = opacities present, few in number.	1 = opacities present, few in number.
2 = numerous opacities, lung markings visible.	2 = numerous opacities, lung markings partly obscured.
3 = very numerous opacities, lung markings obscured.	3 = very numerous opacities, lung markings totally obscured.

Large opacities

A = a single opacity with greatest diameter > 1 cm but < 5 cm or several opacities each > 1 cm, the sum of whose greatest diameters < 5 cm.

B = one or more opacities larger or more numerous than in category A but whose combined area < the area of the right upper zone.

C = as B, but the combined area > area of right upper zone.

*q and r are now used instead of m and n of the previous classification.

pneumoconioses and results from the inhalation of iron dust (atomic no. 26) as iron oxide fume in iron and steel foundries, in rolling mills, during the mining and crushing of iron ores and during grinding and welding operations. The radiological changes disappear when exposure ceases. The inhalation of iron oxide and silver produces the condition known as argyrosiderosis.

Stannosis, caused by deposits of tin (atomic no. 50) in the lungs, is much rarer than siderosis. The opacities in stannosis are much denser than those seen in siderosis and the hilar lymph nodes often stand out, due to the deposition of tin within them. Exposure to tin dust may occur during the handling of the ore, when it is crushed and during the operations of changing and raking out the refinery furnaces. Tin fume will be encountered during any process which involves the molten metal.

Other causes of benign pneumoconiosis include calcium (atomic no. 20) and, rarely, barium (baritosis, atomic no. 56), antimony (atomic no. 51), chromite (atomic no. 22), zirconium (atomic no. 40), and cerium (atomic no. 58). The shadows seen in baritosis are denser even than those in stannosis, and hilar lymph nodes may be prominent. The deposits in the lungs disappear when exposure is discontinued.

FIBROTIC PNEUMOCONIOSIS

Silicosis

Silicosis is the most important and best known of this group of diseases. In considering the disease care must be taken to differentiate between free silica (SiO_2) and silicates which are the salts formed by the combination of silica and basic materials such as calcium oxide and magnesium oxide. Nonfibrous silicates do not harm the lungs unless they contain free silica.

In nature, free silica occurs in flint and quartz and is extremely dangerous. The dust from newly fractured flint is more dangerous than old dust. Natural noncrystalline silica (diatomaceous earth) is relatively nonfibrogenic although after heating it is converted into highly active forms. The most dangerous forms of silica are those produced by heating. At temperatures of between 800–1000°C, tridymite is formed and between 1100–1400°C, cristobalite is produced.

Because of the multitude of uses to which silicaceous rocks have been put, silicosis has acquired a great many colloquial names. For example, the disease has been known at one time or another as dust consumption, grinders' rot, masons' disease, miners' phthisis, potters' rot and stonemasons' disease. Improved methods of dust control and substitution with other materials have resulted in a great decline in the incidence of silicosis although sporadic outbreaks still occur. Substitution has occurred in three principal areas. Artificial abrasives have replaced silica in grinding wheels, calcined alumina replaced ground flint in which pottery was embedded for firing in about 1937 in the pottery industry, and sand has been prohibited for use in blasting operations, being replaced by corundum or silicon carbide.

Signs and symptoms: The principal complaints are of breathlessness and cough but it is important to remember that there may be no symptoms even in those whose chest X-rays show alarming changes. The cough varies in severity and is unproductive unless a secondary infection supervenes. It tends to occur mainly in the mornings but as the disease progresses there may be distressing paroxysms of coughing which are thought to be caused by the stimulation of nerve endings in the trachea and bronchi by silicotic nodules. Breathlessness is first noted during effort and even in severe cases is not present at rest unless some other lung disease is present.

There are remarkably few clinical signs in uncomplicated cases and finger clubbing is not produced nor is there any evidence of central cyanosis.

The complications of silicosis include pulmonary tuberculosis which tends to occur late in life and after moderate or heavy exposure, and right heart failure. Silicosis is the only pneumoconiosis which predisposes to tuberculosis, the onset of which is usually heralded by loss of weight and haemoptysis. Right heart failure is uncommon in silicosis but in those few cases in which it does occur, death is likely from congestive cardiac failure.

Lung function tests: Alterations in pulmonary function are often less severe than the appearances of the chest X-ray might suggest. There is nothing characteristic about the changes but decreases in total lung capacity, in vital capacity, in residual volume and in compliance may be found; there is no evidence of obstructive airways diseases but occasionally there is a slight reduction in gas transfer.

Pathology: The principal lesion is a nodule composed of connective tissue arranged in a whorled pattern (Fig. 6.1a and b). Between the collagen fibres there are collections of dust particles which are usually doubly refracting so that they may readily be seen through a polarizing microscope. The nodules tend to predominate in the upper zones and may coalesce to form confluent masses. The pleura are often adherent and thickened and the lungs may have a gritty feel. Some degree of bronchiectasis is common but emphysema is not a feature of the disease.

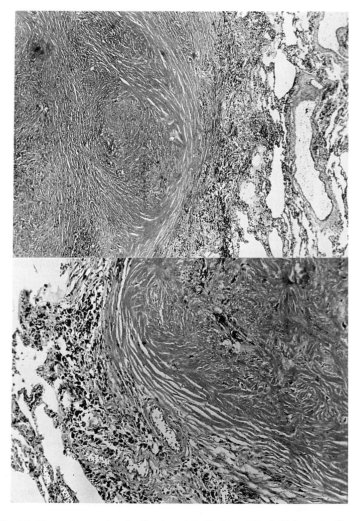

Fig. 6.1. Photomicrographs of a silicotic nodule. Sections stained with haematoxylin and eosin, (a)×39, (b)×98.

Radiography: Discrete rounded nodules of intermediate density are seen throughout the lung fields (Fig. 6.2). These vary in size from 1 to 3 mm in diameter (p and q in ILO classification). As the disease progresses the opacities increase in size and number (ILO category r) and conglomerations appear which eventually develop into large irregular opacities occupying much of the lung field. Calcification in the periphery of the hilar lymph nodes, so-called egg-shell calcification is a feature in some cases (Fig. 6.3). Marked asymetry in the radiological findings is very rare.

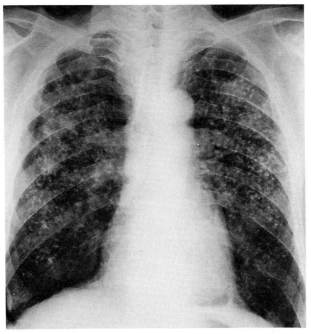

Fig. 6.2. Chest radiograph showing changes of silicosis (category 3.r.) in a flint miller.

Prognosis: Uncomplicated silicosis does not usually cause premature death although in a few individuals the disease progresses and severe respiratory impairment and death follow even if exposure is discontinued. The treatment of silicotuberculosis is generally effective provided that an adequate drug regime is given for a sufficient period. Some cases respond poorly, however, and in them the outlook is poor. The outlook is also poor in those with pulmonary heart disease.

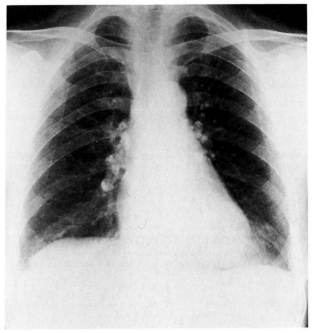

Fig. 6.3. Chest radiograph showing egg-shell calcification in both hilar lymph nodes.

Pathogenesis: There have been a number of theories put forward to explain the fibrogenic effect of free silica. It was at one time thought that minute electrical currents produced by the mechanical deformation of the quartz crystal might damage the fibroblast and initiate fibrosis (the piezoelectric theory) and it has also been considered that crystalline silica might pass into solution in the lung to form silicic acid which would promote fibrosis (the solubility theory). Neither of these theories has many adherents nowadays and most authorities would consider that the initiation of fibrosis results from damage to the alveolar macrophage. Free silica is ingulfed by alveolar macrophages and damages the lysosome membrane. The release of proteolytic enzymes into the cytoplasm causes the death of the macrophage and the further release of the enzymes into the lung where a fibrotic reaction is initiated. It is now becoming accepted that the perpetuation of the fibrosis has an immunological basis. It has been suggested that macrophages exposed to quartz release a factor which stimulates the synthesis of collagen against which an antibody is produced and that this anticollagen antibody actually stimulates fibroblasts to produce more collagen.

Acute silicosis

Acute silicosis is a pulmonary fibrosis, typically with considerable pleural thickening, which develops rapidly as the result of a short exposure to dust containing a high concentration of quartz. The alveolar spaces are filled with an albuminous fluid which is PAS positive, and the appearances are like those in alveolar proteinosis. Silicotic nodules are rarely seen and the condition may thus be differentiated from nodular silicosis of rapid onset in which immature nodules are characteristic.

Symptoms develop quickly, often within a few weeks of exposure to the silicaceous dust. The principal symptom is rapidly progressive dyspnoea with malaise, fatigue, loss of weight, productive cough and pleuritic chest pain. Crepitations may be heard throughout the chest and there is often a pleural rub. Depending on the degree of pleural thickening, breath sounds are diminished or of the bronchial type. Finger clubbing may be present.

The disease is usually fatal within a year of the first appearance of symptoms.

Shaver's disease

This is a disease described in workers processing bauxite (aluminium oxide) in the manufacture of abrasives. The bauxite is fused with iron and coke at high temperatures and fumes of aluminium oxide and silica are evolved. The inhalation of these fumes results in a severe form of pulmonary fibrosis accompanied by emphysema; the symptoms are those of acute silicosis.

On the chest X-ray, a fine reticular pattern of markings is seen, predominantly in the upper zones. The pattern becomes more coarse as the disease progresses. A characteristic feature of the disease is the development of multiple spontaneous pneumothoraces.

Mixed dust fibrosis

This condition results from the inhalation of free silica with substantial amounts of other dusts, most often iron oxides, which reduce its fibrotic activity. The condition occurs in foundry workers, boiler scalers, haematite miners, potters, and in some welders who have worked in foundries.

The lesions produced differ from the classical silicotic nodules in being irregular in shape although they are normally still discrete. The nodules in haematite miners are brick-red in colour, but dark grey in the other groups. In advanced cases, massive fibrosis in the upper zones leads to distortion of the main airways with displacement of the trachea. Tuberculosis is less likely to develop in mixed dust fibrosis than in 'pure' silicosis.

Fibrous silicates

A number of fibrous silicates are used in industry but asbestos is by far the most dangerous. Asbestos is the collective term used to describe some fibrous mineral silicates of which there are two main groups, serpentine and amphibole of differing chemical compositions (Table 6.5).

Asbestos is widely used in industry because of its ability to withstand heat and its excellent insulating properties. Asbestos-cement manufacture consumes the greatest quantity of the fibre and this is followed by the manufacture of floor tiles. An important use is as a component of brake-pads and clutch plates. Of the various forms of asbestos, chrysotile accounts for over 90 per cent of world production. Crocidolite and amosite are next in importance and the remaining forms have a very limited use. In Great Britain the use of crocidolite has been greatly restricted because of its association with malignant mesothelomia but this is not so in other countries of Western Europe, nor in the USA or Japan.

Table 6.5. Classification and chemical composition of asbestos

Serpentine Group	
Chrysotile (white asbestos)	$(OH)_6Mg_6Si_4O_{11}.H_2O$
Amphibole Group	
Actinolite	$Ca(MgFe)_3(SiO_3)_4.xH_2O$
Amosite (brown asbestos)	$(Fe.Mg)SiO_3.1.5\%H_2O$
Anthophyllite	$(Mg.Fe)_7Si_8O_{22}(OH)_2$
Crocidolite (blue asbestos)	$NaFe(SiO_3)_2FeSiO_3.xH_2O$
Tremolite	$Ca_2Mg_5Si_8O_{22}(OH)_2$

Inhalation of asbestos may give rise to several separate conditions:
1   Asbestosis, by which is meant fibrosis of the lung with or without pleural fibrosis;
2   Benign pleural disease;

3   Bronchial carcinoma and
4   Malignant mesothelioma.

Bronchial carcinoma and mesothelioma are discussed in Chapter 8 and will not be considered here.

Asbestosis

Asbestos is a form of diffuse interstitial fibrosis and it is most important to understand that it is a dose-related disease. A clear linear relationship between increasing dust exposure and the development of asbestosis has been demonstrated and only those who have been heavily exposed for a long time are in danger of contracting it. The fibrosis which is seen is typically distributed subpleurally over the lower half of the lungs. The pulmonary pleura may be thickened, invariably so when lung fibrosis is advanced, although the degree of fibrosis in the pleura does not always match that in the lungs. Bronchiectasis is found in a few cases in areas of severe fibrosis but emphysema is uncommon and the hilar lymph nodes are not enlarged. The typical microscopic picture is one of fibrosing alveolitis with gradual obliteration of the air spaces by collagen. Asbestos bodies are seen in the areas of fibrosis and in the sputum (Fig. 6.4).

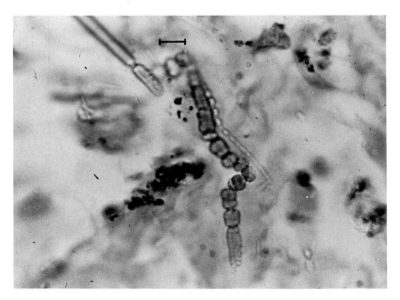

Fig. 6.4. Photomicrograph of an asbestos body in the sputum of a man with asbestosis. Note the characteristic beaded appearance. Bar = 10μ.

Asbestos bodies are long structures, up to 80 μm in length, and they consist of asbestos fibres coated with layers of iron-containing protein which imparts a golden-yellow or brown colour to them. The protein coat is usually fragmented so that the asbestos bodies tend to have a beaded appearance. They are readily detected in sections of lung tissue as they stain blue with Perl's reagent.

It is important to realize that whilst the presence of asbestos bodies in the sputum is indicative of past exposure to asbestos it does not signify proof of asbestosis.

Symptoms of asbestosis: The symptoms of asbestosis are insidious and there is a variable latent period between their appearance and first exposure. Dyspnoea is the first symptom to be noted. At first moderate, the breathlessness increases in severity and patients find difficulty in taking a deep breath because of the reduced compliance of the lungs. This is not unique to asbestosis but occurs in any form of interstitial fibrosis. The degree of breathlessness may be out of all proportion to the changes seen on the chest film and may be severe even when there are few physical signs in the chest.

Cough is absent during the early stages but as the disease advances, becomes much more common. There is usually little sputum. Chest

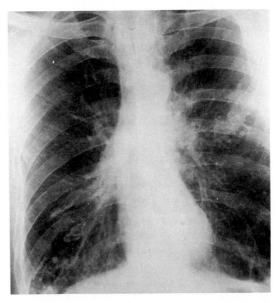

Fig. 6.5. Chest radiograph showing changes due to asbestosis with pleural plaques.

pain is not a feature but most patients with severe disease complain of lassitude.

Physical signs: Signs in the chest are few considering the degree of disability. In advanced cases there is an impairment of chest expansion affecting particularly the lower part of the chest and this is a useful measure by which to screen men at work. Persistent crepitations heard during inspiration are discovered early in the disease, often before there are any changes on X-ray and this is an important sign of pathological change. Finger clubbing is frequently present.

Radiography: Abnormal radiographic signs in asbestosis are more common in the lower zones than elsewhere (Fig. 6.5). This contrasts with the situation in silicosis and coal miners' pneumoconiosis where the changes are more common in the upper zones. The radiological signs are those of diffuse interstitial fibrosis (ILO categories s, t or u) with fine punctate mottling. A cystic or honey-comb appearance may develop but the cystic spaces remain small, usually less than 5 mm. The costophrenic angles become obliterated and the cardiac outline becomes blurred and there is evidence of pleural thickening.

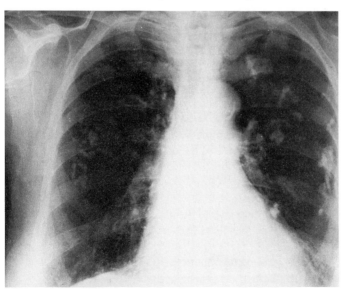

Fig. 6.6. Chest radiograph showing pleural plaques due to asbestos exposure. The patient, a female journalist, had never worked in industry but was brought up near an asbestos mine in Canada.

Pleural plaques are often overlooked unless they are calcified when they are seen as irregular shadows of patchy density. They may be seen in the absence of other evidence of asbestosis and in those with no history of an occupational exposure to asbestos (Fig. 6.6).

Pulmonary function: The earliest abnormality in lung function in cases of asbestosis is decreased compliance and this can be noted before there are any signs or symptoms of the disease. Measuring compliance is difficult under routine conditions and so in the monitoring of asbestos workers the vital capacity (VC) is used. A consistent reduction in VC in the absence of significant airways obstruction or any other chronic chest disease is a good indication that compliance is reduced and is the most sensitive routine test by which to detect the effects of asbestos exposure. Other functional abnormalities which are noted include reduction in total lung capacity and reduction in diffusing capacity for carbon monoxide.

Pathogenesis: The pathogenesis of asbestosis is not fully understood although it is known that asbestos fibres are cytotoxic; this can be demonstrated *in vivo* by their capacity to haemolyse red cells. The fibrogenic property of asbestos fibres is determined by their length, those which are longer than $10-20$ μm are fibrogenic whereas shorter fibres are not. Long fibres are incompletely ingested by macrophages and they damage the cell membrane allowing the release of enzymes and other constituents which may initiate the fibrotic process. Long fibres are also poorly cleared from the lung and, since they are not broken down by the macrophages, their potential to harm the cells is increased. As with silicosis, it is probable that immunological responses also have a part to play in the development of the fibrosis. After the ingestion of asbestos fibres the surface of the macrophage shows an increase in the number of receptors for both the C3 component of complement and for IgG antibodies. Asbestos fibres also activate both the classical and the alternative complement pathways. These findings suggest that the activation of complement and the alteration in the antigenic properties of the macrophage may have an important role to play in the development of asbestosis.

The earlier observation that there was an association between HLA antigens and asbestosis has not been confirmed nor have reports that the number of T suppressor cells is diminished. We have not heard the last of the immunology of asbestosis, however.

Treatment: Once established, asbestosis generally progresses to produce some degree of respiratory disability. The time scale is variable, however, and susceptible individuals may become respiratory cripples within 2 or 3 years of developing symptoms whereas others live into their sixties or seventies, finally dying from a cause unconnected with asbestos. Removing men from contact with asbestos does not materially alter the rate of progress of the disease.

There is no treatment which can be offered except supportive measures as required.

Neighbourhood cases: Cases of asbestosis have been reported in persons living close to asbestos mines or asbestos-using factories even though they themselves have no occupational exposure. There is no doubt that residents living near factories were subjected to a considerable degree of contamination in the past, but modern measures of control have eliminated this hazard in the United Kingdom. Another source of hazard to the public was from dust carried out by workmen on their clothes, but regulations now forbid the wearing of work clothes outside the factory. Asbestos building materials if not properly sealed may become friable and release dust into the atmosphere and thus constitute a risk. Similarly, the demolition of buildings with asbestos in their fabric may release dust to the atmosphere if the proper precautions are not taken.

Prevention: The Asbestos Regulation which came into force in 1970 controlled the use of asbestos and they have been supplemented by the Asbestos (Licensing) Regulations of 1983. These regulations prohibit anyone carrying out work with asbestos insulation or asbestos coatings unless they hold a licence issued by the Health and Safety Executive. Furthermore all those who are to be engaged on work with asbestos insulations or coatings must be medically examined before they begin the work and at intervals of not more than 2 years thereafter unless their work is of short duration (less than 2 hours in total) or they are engaged solely in the collection of samples or air monitoring.

It is likely that the use of asbestos spraying will be banned in the near future and asbestos is also likely to be banned for most thermal and acoustic insulation purposes. Crocidolite is no longer used and the use of amosite is discouraged. As from 1 August 1984, there are new control limits for asbestos in the air. The concentration of dusts containing crocidolite or amosite must not exceed 0.2 fibres/ml and that of other types of asbestos must not exceed 0.5 fibres/ml when calculated in relation to a 4 hour reference period.

Benign pleural disease

A number of pleural syndromes may be seen in those who have been exposed to asbestos including pleural plaques, pleural thickening and pleural effusion. Pleural plaques are elevated areas which consist of collagen fibres; they tend to become calcified in those parts of the lesion where the collagen has degenerated. They are found on the parietal pleura, and they tend to be more frequent on the posterolateral and basal parts, and on the central tendon of the diaphragm. Their presence indicates exposure to asbestos or to some other mineral fibres; they are not diagnostic of asbestosis. Pleural plaques are commmon in some parts of eastern Europe and Asia Minor where mineral fibres such as zeolite, but not asbestos, may be present in the environment.

Diffuse thickening of the pleura may be noted with or without pleural plaques. The costophrenic angles may be obliterated and thickening of the parietal pleura in the inter-lobar fissures may be the only radiological evidence of exposure to asbestos. Thickening of the visceral pleura may on rare occasions produce folding of the lung producing an appearance which mimics that of a tumour.

Pleural effusions are the most troublesome of the benign pleural conditions which may afflict asbestos workers. They may be asymptomatic but they are often accompanied by pleuritic pain and occasionally by dyspnoea. There may also be a slight fever. The effusion is usually small in volume but it is often blood stained, a feature which causes much alarm and fears that a mesothelioma may be present. In some cases diffuse pleural thickening may develop after the fluid has been absorbed and this may cause a restrictive lung defect of such severity that pleurectomy is required.

OTHER FIBROUS SILICATES

Talc

Talc is an hydrated magnesium silicate with the formula $Mg_3Si_4O_{10}(OH)_2$. It also contains calcium, aluminium and iron in variable amounts and may contain other minerals, including asbestos and quartz. Three clinical syndromes which have been reported to follow the inhalation of talc are:

1 an irregular nodular fibrosis
2 interstitial fibrosis with talc bodies similar to asbestos bodies
3 foreign body granulomata

The inhalation of pure talc gives rise to the formation of granulomata, but the first lesions are probably due to the inhalation of contaminating minerals such as quartz or asbestos whose action is modified by the talc. Any or all of the three lesions may be present in an exposed population. The radiological changes, which are confined mainly to the lower and mid-zones, are similar to those found in asbestosis. Thus fibrotic change is the major feature, and calcified pleural plaques may also be present, usually bilateral in distribution. In addition, there may be signs of pleural adhesions and enlargement of the hilar shadow. There are no nodules, such as might be found in silicosis.

Symptoms develop gradually after prolonged exposure. Fifteen or twenty years is the usual time scale. Dyspnoea and cough are most frequently noted. The disease usually progresses slowly and does not significantly alter life expectancy except in those cases who develop massive fibrosis or diffuse interstitial fibrosis. There is no predisposition to tuberculosis or mesothelioma. There has been some suggestion that the incidence of bronchial carcinoma may be higher than expected in talc workers but this is not a generally accepted view.

Sillimanite minerals

The sillimanite minerals, andalusite, kyanite and sillimanite are all forms of alumium silicate ($Al_2O_3.SiO_2$). They have the properties of being extremely resistant to acids and alkalis and of being able to withstand very high temperatures. They are used mainly to make laboratory porcelain, spark plug casings and refractory bricks.

At most, these minerals cause only mild fibrosis and few reported cases of pneumoconiosis have been convincingly shown to be due to their sole action.

Man-made mineral fibres

Man-made mineral fibres are used increasingly to replace asbestos for thermal and acoustic insulation. There are three main groups, slag wools, rock wools and glass wools and filaments; all are amorphous silicates. The mineral wools are made from melts of natural limestone rock or smelter slags sometimes with the addition of wollastonite or kaolinite. Glass fibres are made either from borosilicate or calcioalumina silicate glass. The fibres are commonly coated with a binder which is a biologically inert resin but may be mineral oil. Unlike asbestos fibres which tend to split longitudinally into particles with a smaller diameter than the parent fibre, man-made fibres split transversely to produce short fragments with the same diameter.

There are no convincing reports of respiratory effects following exposure to man-made mineral fibres nor have any radiographic changes been consistently noted. There is some concern that these fibres may cause bronchial carcinoma; they are not thought to cause mesothelioma. The results of a recent large scale epidemiological study in Europe do suggest that there was a slightly increased risk in the past but with present very low levels of exposure, the risk has probably disappeared.

NON-FIBROUS SILICATES

This group includes mica, kaolin and other clays, fullers' earth and bentonite.

Mica

The family of mica minerals comprises muscovite (potassium alumium silicate), biotite (a complex silicate containing magnesium aluminium, potassium and iron) and vermiculite (magnesium-aluminium silicates derived from biotite).

There is little in the way of firm evidence to show that any of these minerals causes pulmonary fibrosis although a few workers exposed to mica dust have been found to have minor changes on X-ray consistent with pneumoconiosis.

Kaolin (China clay)

China clays are predominantly composed of hydrous aluminium silicate ($2H_2O.Al_2O_3.2SiO_2$), also known as kaolinite. Other than as the main ingredient of china clay, it is used as a filler in rubber, paints, plastics and papers, and high purity kaolin is used medicinally.

Pneumoconiosis affects only a small minority of men exposed and then only after a prolonged period, and it is by no means certain whether the symptoms are due entirely to kaolin or to contaminants such as quartz. The lesions reported include nodular fibrosis, sometimes massive fibrosis and mild diffuse interstitial fibrosis, whilst reported symptoms include breathlessness with cough and sputum.

Non-kaolin clays

These clays contain a higher proportion of quartz than china clays, hence pneumoconiosis is rather more frequent and of the silicotic, nodular type.

Fullers' earth and bentonite

Fullers' earth is a clay so named because of its one-time use to remove grease from wool and cloth, a process known as fulling. It is a fine-grained, absorbent clay composed mainly of calcium montmorillonite. Quartz is found in some deposits and this may produce silicotic lesions in those working or mining it. Other radiographic changes which have been found include small, discrete opacities of low density, especially in the upper zones, which occasionally coalesce. This form of pneumoconiosis is essentially benign and does not shorten life expectancy. Bentonite clays contain 85 per cent or more of montmorillonite and are harmless unless they contain quartz.

COAL MINERS' PNEUMOCONIOSIS

This disease occurs in miners exposed to coal dust whether at the coal face or elsewhere. The pathological lesions which develop are caused by the inhalation of carbon, and similar lesions may develop in workers exposed to other forms of carbon. The development of the disease is dependent upon the amount of dust inhaled and the duration of exposure. It is distinct from silicosis although mixed dust fibrosis is found in coal miners who have also been exposed to silica.

Simple pneumoconiosis

The early lesions are small discrete macules of dust found mainly in the upper zones. They are found to be concentrated around the respiratory bronchioles and are enmeshed in reticulin fibres. Collagen is found in early lesions but later fibrotic changes ensue to produce black fibrous nodules. Pseudo-asbestos bodies are sometimes found in the dust-containing lesions. They consist of spicules of coal or carbon and a covering of iron-containing protein which gives a positive Prussian blue reaction.

Progressive massive fibrosis (PMF)

Large black fibrotic masses consisting of coal dust and bundles of collagen occur in some cases. These lesions tend to concentrate in the upper and mid zones but there are many exceptions to the rule. When near the periphery, the overlying pleura is involved and may become fibrotic and adherent to the parietal layer. A lesion is defined as PMF when its diameter is greater than 3 cm. Necrosis and cavitation of the lesions are well known complications.

Caplan's syndrome

Caplan's syndrome is a modified form of pneumoconiosis found in association with rheumatoid arthritis. The majority of cases occur in coal miners, but the disease may be found in men in a wide variety of dusty trades. The nodules in the lung are scattered irregularly through the lung and are up to 2 cm in diameter. They have a characteristic concentric appearance with alternating laminae of coal-dust and necrotic collagen. Cavitation is common and sometimes the nodules aggregate to form structures which closely resemble a collection of silicotic nodules. Coal-dust macules are typically absent but where they are in evidence, they are the same as in non-rheumatoid miners.

Symptoms: Simple pneumoconiosis is asymptomatic. In PMF symptoms may be trivial or such as to cause severe disability. There is little correlation between radiological findings and the severity of symptoms. In most miners cough and sputum are more related to the development of bronchitis which seems to be due to coal dust exposure, aided in many instances by smoking. In some cases of PMF a severe unproductive cough brought on by effort is a distressing feature of the disease. If a massive fibrotic lesion ruptures into a bronchus large amounts of jet-black sputum are brought up and this may continue for several days.

Signs: Coal pneumoconiosis has no characteristic signs although wheezes and rhonchi may be heard throughout the lung field. In patients with PMF the trachea may be displaced by lesions in the upper zones. Large PMF may be accompanied by signs of right heart failure. Finger clubbing is extremely rare.

In patients with Caplan's syndrome, signs of pleural effusion may indicate the onset, or the exacerbation, of the symptoms of rheumatoid arthritis.

Radiology: The earlier radiological signs to appear are a few small, ill-defined opacities in the mid and upper zones. Opacities of different size may be present in one film but most come into the q category. As simple pneumoconiosis progresses the opacities come to be found more or less equally distributed throughout the lung fields (Fig. 6.7).

PMF opacities (Fig. 6.8) are also usually seen in the upper zones and may be unilateral or bilateral, symmetrical or asymmetrical. These appearances are usually set on a ground of simple pneumoconiosis but this is not invariable. The shape of the opacities in PMF varies considerably and cavitation is indicated by an area of translucency within an opacity.

In a few cases 'egg-shell' calcification of the hilar lymph nodes is seen, similar to that which is seen in silicosis. It happens more frequently in conjunction with PMF than with simple pneumoconiosis.

The dense, round opacities in Caplan's syndrome are irregularly

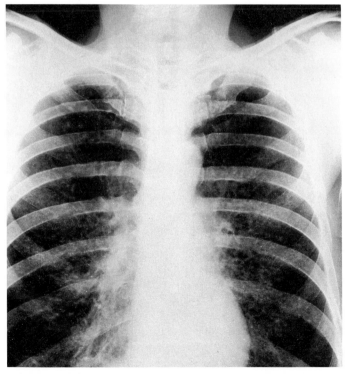

Fig. 6.7. Chest radiograph showing the changes of simple pneumoconiosis in a coal miner who had worked 26 years underground. Changes are in categories 2.q. and 2.s.

scattered throughout the lung fields and are usually few in number. There are normally no signs of simple pneumoconiosis.

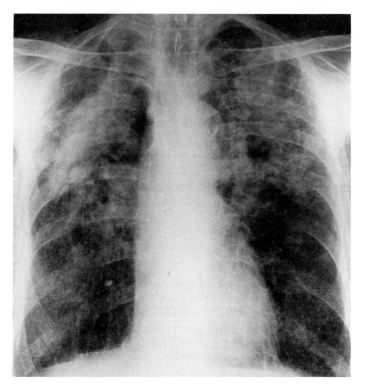

Fig. 6.8. Chest radiograph showing PMF and simple pneumoconiosis in a miner who had worked underground for 30 years. Changes are in category 3.q./C.

Exposure to coal dust and emphysema: For some years there has been a debate as to whether exposure to coal dust predisposes to the development of emphysema. The most recent information shows that there is a clear relationship between measured exposure to respirable coal dust and both FEV_1 and decline in FEV_1 over time. Postmortem studies have also shown that miners have a higher prevalence of emphysema than controls and that the more coal dust present in the lung, the greater the likelihood that the lung will show centriacinar emphysema.

RESPIRATORY FUNCTION IN OCCUPATIONAL LUNG DISEASES

Respiratory function tests are being used increasingly to monitor men exposed to dust and other materials known to affect the lungs. The tests most often used for routine screening purposes are the measurement of forced expiratory volume (FEV), usually the volume expelled in one second (FEV_1), the forced vital capacity (FVC) and the vital capacity (VC). These are all measurements which can be made using a simple, portable respirometer and are thus, most suitable for use in industry.

Three broad categories of impairment in lung function can be recognized.

1. Airways obstruction

Asthma, bronchitis and emphysema produce some narrowing of the airways with a resultant obstruction to air flow, predominantly during expiration. In asthma this is usually reversible but only rarely so in bronchitis and emphysema. As a result FEV_1 values are low but VC is

Table 6.6. Patterns of change in lung function tests in occupational lung diseases

	VC	FVC	FEV_1	Gas exchange
Silicosis	↓↓ (in advanced cases)			↓
Acute silicosis	↓↓	↓↓		↓↓↓
Coal pneumoconiosis				
Simple	↓	↓		↓
PMF	↓↓			↓↓
Asbestosis	↓↓	↓↓	↓↓ (FEV_1:FVC greater than normal)	↓↓
Chronic beryllium disease	↓	↓	↓	↓↓
Extrinsic allergic alveolitis	↓↓			↓↓
Byssinosis			↓↓ (progressive fall during working day)	
Asthma	↓	↓↓	↓↓	

↓ Slightly reduced   ↓↓ Reduced   ↓↓↓ Greatly reduced

larger than FVC because forced expiration increases the degree of narrowing in the airways.

2. Reduced compliance

A reduction in compliance is found in those diseases which produce diffuse interstitial fibrosis. The lungs are unable to expand fully and there is a resultant decrease in VC and FVC. Asbestosis is the most important occupational disease in this class and the VC is an excellent screening test for lung damage in asbestos workers.

3. Impairment of gas exchange

Gas exchange is impaired whenever ventilation is reduced relative to blood flow, either locally or generally, or vice versa. It is also impaired by diseases which affect the architecture of the alveoli such as diffuse interstitial fibrosis and granulomatous lung disorders.

Tests of gas exchange need to be conducted in a laboratory and on this account are not suitable to be used for screening purposes.

A summary of the changes in respiratory function seen in the occupational lung diseases is shown in Table 6.6.

CHAPTER 7/DISEASES OF
THE SKIN

OCCUPATIONAL DERMATITIS

The prevalence of occupational dermatitis is high in all industrialized countries. In Great Britain more days are lost as a result of skin disease than from all the other prescribed diseases put together. In men, approximately 650,000 working days a year are lost, and for women, approximately 200,000 days a year are lost. These figures are some indication of the cost to the community, but they give no indication of the amount of misery and discomfort experienced by the patients, much of which could be avoided by proper precautionary measures.

The agents which cause skin lesions are many and varied but can be divided into five classes as follows:
1   Mechanical factors, such as friction, pressure and trauma,
2   Physical factors including heat, cold, electricity, sunlight and radiation,
3   Chemical agents, both organic and inorganic,
4   Plants and their products, resins and lacquers, and
5   Other biological agents such as infective organisms, insects and mites.

The relative importance of each of these naturally depends on the occupation being considered, but in general, chemical agents are by far the greatest cause of occupational skin disorders.

1. Mechanical factors

Mechanical factors give rise to cuts and abrasions which may become secondarily infected. Repeated trauma produces callosities, the sites of which are determined by the particular occupation and will often identify a man's job to the knowledgeable observer.

Callosities may develop at specific points of pressure between the skin and any tool or instrument which is being used constantly. Occupations in which one might expect to find them thus include carpenters, painters, cobblers, dressmakers, floor sweepers and so on. In other workers, the callosities develop on the whole palmar surface of the hand in response to general trauma. The callosities are of no pathological significance but rather, they have a function to protect underlying tissues.

2. Physical factors

Heat may affect the skin by causing excessive perspiration which softens the protective horny layers. When combined with frictional stress, it can produce intertrigo, the so-called heat rashes of furnace men, stokers and others who work under hot conditions.

Cold injuries to the skin include chilblains, and if associated with damp or wet conditions may produce trench foot in extreme cases. In our climate, extremes of temperature are unusual so that frost bite is not a condition which is likely to be encountered.

Burns resulting from accidents at work are a real hazard in industry, although they rarely result from electrical accidents. They may occur from an overenthusiastic exposure to the sun on the part of those whose work takes them outdoors. Prolonged exposure to sunlight can undoubtedly be a factor in the production of skin cancer. Exposure to ionizing radiation also has the dual effect of burning and inducing malignant change, but adequate safety measures should ensure that neither is seen nowadays.

3. Chemical agents

These are responsible for the great bulk of occupational skin disease and they act either as primary irritants or sensitizers (or both).

Primary irritants

Primary irritants are agents which produce lesions by direct action at the site of contact. Their speed of action depends on their concentration and the length of time for which they are in contact with the skin. Their effects are caused by chemical reactions with the skin; by degreasing or dehydrating; by denaturing proteins in the skin, or by disturbing the osmotic pressure of the cells in the skin. Alkali seems to cause most skin trouble, but the list of primary irritants is enormous and constantly on the increase as the number of chemicals in use rises steadily year by year. Some of the more important primary irritants are listed in Table 7.1 but it must be emphasized that this list is far from being complete.

Table 7.1. Principal primary skin irritants in industry.*

Alkalis

Inorganic

Alkaline sulphides	Barium hydrate and carbonate
Sodium hydrate, carbonate, silicate and metasilicate	Calcium oxide, hydrate carbonate and cyanamide
Potassium hydrate and carbonate	Trisodium phosphate
Ammonium hydrate and carbonate	

Organic

Ethanolamines	Methylamine

Acids

Inorganic

Arsenious	Hydrofluoric
Chloroplatinic	Hydrofluosilic
Chlorosulphonic	Nitric
Chromic	Perchloric
Hydriotic	Phosphoric
Hydrobromic	Sulphuric
Hydrochloric	

Organic

Acetic	Maleic
Carbolic	Metanilic
Cresylic	Oxalic
Formic	Salicylic
Lactic	

Elements and their salts

Antimony and salts	Mercuric salts
Arsenic and salts	Nickel salts
Chromium and alkaline chromates	Zinc chloride
Copper sulphate	Silver nitrate
Copper cyanide	

Solvents

Petroleum solvents	Turpentine
Coal tar solvents	Terpenes
Chlorinated hydrocarbons	Carbon bisulphide
Esters	Alcohols
Ketones	

Acne producers

Petroleum oils	Chloronaphthalenes
Cutting oils	Chlorodiphenyls
Pitch	Chlorodiphenyloxides
Tar	Solid chlorobenzols
Paraffin	Solid chlorophenols

*From Schwartz L., Tulipan L. and Birmingham D.J., *Occupational Diseases of the Skin*, Kingston, London, 1957.

Sensitizers

Many chemicals do not have a primary irritant effect, instead, contact
with them results in a type of cell-mediated hypersensitivity reaction.
The resultant lesion is referred to as contact dermatitis. The sensitizing
chemical passes through the epidermal barrier and reacts with a protein
to produce a hapten against which antibodies are formed. Once the
antibodies are produced, the skin reaction will occur whenever the
hapten is formed.

Table 7.2. Principal skin sensitizers in industry

Dye intermediates

Aniline and compounds	Naphthalene and compounds
Chloro compounds	Benzidine and compounds
Nitro compounds	Benzanthrone and compounds
Acridine and compounds	Naphthylamines

Dyes

Paraphenylendiamine	Metanil yellow
Aniline black	Brilliant indigo, 4 G.
Paramido phenol	Erio black
Chrysoidine	Hydron blue
Bismarck brown	Indanthrene violet, R. R.
Nigrosine	Ionamine, A. S.
Amido-azo-toluene	Pyrogene violet brown
Amido-azo-benzene	Orange Y
Crystal and methyl violet	Safranine
Malachite green	Sulphanthrene pink
Auramine	Rosaniline

Photographic developers

Paraphenylendiamine	Pyrogallol
Hydroquinone	Bichromates
Para-amido-phenol	Paraformaldehyde
Metol	

Rubber accelerators and anti-oxidants

Hexamethylene tetramine	Para toluidine
Guanidines	Ortho toluidine
Mercapto benzo thiazole	Triethyl tri-methyl triamine
Tetromethyl thiuram monosulphide and disulphide	

Insecticides

Creosote	*Arsenic compounds
Nicotine	*Fluorides
Tar	*Lime
Pyrethrum	Rotenone
*Mercury compounds	Thiocyanates

*Phenol compounds
*Petroleum distillates

Organic phosphates

Oils

Cutting oils (the inhibitor or
   antiseptic they contain)
Coning oils (cellosolves, eugenols)
Sulphonated oils
Linseed oil

*Mustard oil
Coconut oil
*Cashew nut oil
Tung oil
Essential oils of plants and flowers

Natural resins

Pine rosin
Wood rosin
Burgundy pitch

Japanese lacquer
Dammar
Copal

Synthetic resins

Alkyd
Vinyl
Acrylic
Phenol formaldehyde
Urea formaldehyde
Melamine formaldehyde
Sulphonamide formaldehyde
Chloro-naphthalenes

Chlorobenzols
Chlorodiphenyls
Chlorophenols
Cumaron
Epoxies
Polyesters
Urethane

Coal tar and its direct derivatives

Acridine
Anthracene
Phenanthrene
Carbazole
Pyridine

Fluorene
Naphthalene
*Phenol
*Cresol

Explosives

Trinitrotoluene
Trinitromethylnitramine (Tetryl)
Fulminate of mercury
Hexanitrodiphenylamine
Dinitrophenol
Dinitrotoluol

Lead styphnate
Ammonium nitrate
Sodium nitrate
Potassium nitrate
Picric acid and picrates
Sensol

Plasticizers

Propylene stearate
Butyl cellosolve stearate
Diamyl naphthalene
Dibutyl tin laurate
Dioctylphthalate

Methyl cellosolve oleate
Methyl phthalylethylglycol
Phenylsalicylate
Stearic acid
Triblycol di (2, ethyl butyrate)

Others

Enzymes derives from *B. subtilis*

---

*Compounds which also act as primary irritants From Schwartz L., Tulipan L. and
Birmingham D.J., *Occupational Diseases of the Skin*. Kingston, London, 1957.

The list of sensitizers is again formidable and some primary irritants such as the bichromates, the phenols, and formaldehyde are also sensitizers. Table 7.2 shows some of the more important sensitizers. These chemicals have in common a great affinity for keratin with which they form haptens.

Clinical picture

Whether the skin lesion is produced by primary irritants or by sensitizers, the changes are essentially the same, although it should be noted that sensitivity rashes may occur away from the area in contact with the sensitizer. The first change to be noted is erythema often accompanied by irritation. Following this, vesicles are formed, which burst to produce a red weeping lesion. Healing is associated with crusting and the damping down of the inflammatory reaction.

The organic arsenic and mercury compounds are powerful vesicants and other chemicals such as chrome, alkalis, washing soda, brine and lime cause ulceration. The ulcers are often sufficiently characteristic to be identified with a fair degree of precision. Mercury fulminate causes small necrotic lesions known as powder holes and a more generalized, pruritic, papular lesion called fulminate itch.

The site of the lesion will depend upon which parts of the skin have been in contact with the pathogenic chemical and this alone may give the clue to its identity. Often the easiest forms to recognize are those which occur on the fingers or hands due to the wearing of rubber gloves. It is not always so easy to identify the substances which are responsible, however, if only because many men will not know the chemicals with which they have been in contact, or know them only by trade names. Again, the man's description of his job may often give no clue to the chemicals which he handles. The task of identification is comparatively easy if he comes into contact with only one chemical or group of chemicals, mineral oil, epoxy resins, and so on. It is always helpful to ask whether any of his colleagues have had skin trouble, since the diagnosis of occupational skin disease is made much more certain if fellow workers have experienced similar troubles.

Once the field has been narrowed down the responsible agent (or agents) can be sought through patch testing. Patch testing is not infallible and indeed may sometimes be misleading. It may sometimes exacerbate the condition and should only be done by experts. Despite the drawbacks of the technique, it should always be attempted, since if the cause for the dermatitis can be identified, then the patient can be protected from it.

Occupational acne

This common form of occupational dermatitis is caused by oils, pitch and tar, and some chlorinated hydrocarbons. The chloronaphthalenes are the most potent acne producers but the greatest number of cases are caused by exposure to mineral oil.

The chemicals which cause acne have a dual action, plugging the pores of the skin whilst at the same time promoting the production of keratin. The result is the formation of comedomes and cysts, which in the case of exposure to oils is almost always proceded by folliculitis. Inflammatory reactions are the rule when considering acne due to cutting oils; they are the exception in acne due to tar or chlorinated hydrocarbons.

4. Plants and their products

Plants and their products cause dermatitis by virtue of the chemical compounds which they contain. The list of those plants which are harmful is of majestic length. Fortunately the family of plants which is most effective in causing skin lesions, the Anacardiaceae, does not grow in this country. Those which do sometimes give trouble are predominantly members of the Liliaceae and the Primulaceae. Those affected are farmers, gardeners, nurserymen and florists as would be expected.

Tulip finger is a condition found amongst farmers handling bulbs from which the juice is oozing. The lesion is confined around and under the nails although the nail itself is not affected. Painful lesions of the same sort may also occur amongst those picking tulips, daffodils or narcissi and it is thought that lime salts in the sap are here acting as primary irritants, though, of course, almost any plant is liable to produce an idiosyncratic skin reaction in a susceptible individual. In some cases there is an itching, desquamating rash accompanied by fissuring and this is known as lily rash. The incidence of both types of dermatitis shows a marked seasonal variation as would be anticipated, and on occasion has been severe enough to disrupt the flower industry in Cornwall and the Scilly Isles.

The Primulaceae secrete a toxin in the form of a sticky yellowy-green liquid and gardeners and florists are frequently affected by it. The rash typically consists of numerous close-packed shiny red punctiform papules which may coalesce to form small vesicles or large blisters. There is much smarting and itching as an accompaniment. The toxin may be conveyed by other agencies to the affected individual. For example, cow men have been affected by touching the udders of cows which have passed over cowslips picking up the toxin as they do so.

Of all the species, the hot house *Primula obconica* is the most irritant and affects something like half of those coming into contact with it.

Toxic woods

Dermatitis from woods is frequent amongst carpenters, wood machinists, workers in wood yards, cabinet makers, shipbuilders and furniture makers. The culpable substances can be the saw dust, the sap and the polishings, or the oil of the wood. It is usually imported woods, or woods not handled before which cause trouble. Some wood dusts can produce respiratory symptoms in susceptible individuals (see Chapter 6).

Woods usually produce a sensitivity reaction so that the worker becomes affected several days after beginning to work with a new wood. Most of those affected become desensitized, but there is a minority of men who remain highly sensitized. The reactions occur when the wood is in a certain stage of drying out and so outbreaks of dermatitis occur when consignments in the appropriate condition are used. Once the consignments are finished, the outbreak ceases.

Most cases have minimal symptoms with a papulo-vesicular rash on the hands and arms which clears quickly with treatment. In some cases, however, more severe symptoms may be produced. *Gonioma kamassi*, known more often as Kamassi boxwood, will cause systemic effects in susceptible individuals due to the liberation of an alkaloid which has curare-like effects. The myocardium is affected and a marked brady-cardia is produced. Those affected become subject to a marked languor with mental dullness in addition. There may be repeated episodes of an influenzal-like illness. This wood was at one time widely used in the manufacture of shuttles for the cotton industry. It had to be discon-tinued from this use, however, because of the epidemic lethargy induced in the men who made the shuttles. Iroko wood, which is used as a substitute for teak, has also been known to produce symptoms resem-bling influenza, particularly if the wood is badly seasoned. Asthmatic symptoms may also occur. This skin rash is intensely irritant and is accompanied by facial oedema, conjunctivitis and blepharospasm in some cases.

Many other woods will produce dermatitis but good preventive measures will minimize the hazard. These include exhaust ventilation to remove dust, and the provision of protective clothing and respirators where appropriate.

5. Other biological agents

Grain itch, barley itch, copra itch and grocers' itch are all varieties of dermatitis caused by mites. Grain itch and barley itch occur in men handling cargoes of grain infested with *Pediculoides ventricosus*, a mite which normally feeds on the grain moth. The skin lesion develops after a period of 12 to 16 hours and consists of papules, vesicles, pustules and urticarial wheals on the face, neck, arms and trunk. Copra itch is found to occur in dock workers handling copra infested with *Tryoglyphus longior* which causes intensely irritant papules to develop after an incubation period of 1 day. The cheese mite is of the same family and it causes skin eruptions in grocers amongst others, hence the eponym. Another of the family lives in raw vanilla and attacks those coming into contact with it. Decomposing figs harbour a mite, *Carpoglyphus passularum*, which causes a pruritic rash in handling this fruit. The mite is also found in other fruits such as prunes and dates.

Outbreaks of scabies are well known to occur in camps occupied by soldiers and other groups such as miners and lumberjacks and in any group of people working in closely crowded, unhygienic conditions. It is the lack of hygiene rather than the occupation which predisposes to the infestation. Certain forms of animal scabies, on the other hand, may be found in humans by reason of their work. Thus veterinary practitioners can become infected with the mites that give rise to sarcoptic mange in horses, dogs and cats. Rarely, dairymen are infected by cattle mange and the condition is then known as dairyman's itch. The rash produced is intensely pruritic. In horse mange, which was very common in the days when the horse was the main form of transport, the itching is accompanied by red papules about the size of a pin head. The mite does not propagate in human skin so that the lesions are transitory and the burrows which are typical of the human variant are not found.

Colour changes in the skin

Colour changes in the skin are specific to several occupations. Men handling dyes and other chemicals are especially prone, the colour change being dependent upon the dye, or dyes in use. Men handling chromates develop yellow stains on their hands, so do those employed in the manufacture of TNT and DNB. Picric acid imparts a light yellow colour to the skin whilst tetryl gives it an apricot tint. Those who handle silver nitrate have darkened skin; the photographer's fingers and nails are brown from metol and men handling pitch and tar have black skins. Men who worked for several years in contact with arsenic are often found to have a fine, mottled brown pigmentation, the so-called rain-drop pigmentation. It occurred predominantly on the face and neck but in severe cases, there was an intense bronze colour on the chest, abdomen and back. The argyria of silver workers has already been mentioned in Chapter 2. Most coal miners carry pigmented scars on their bodies due to the impregnation of small cuts and abrasions with coal dust and the same is true of other miners, the ultimate colour of the scar depending on the material being worked. Men chiselling steel are also liable to show the same phenomenon as small chips of metal enter the skin and become oxidized.

Vitiligo

Vitiligo occurs amongst workers handling p-tert-butylphenol (PTBP) which is used in the production of resins which go to make adhesives used in the car industry. The depigmentation has been noted in those manufacturing the raw product and in car workers using the adhesives prepared from it.

The condition is morphologically indistinguishable from true vitiligo but there is no evidence of an autoimmune disorder as in the true condition; those affected do not have an unusual incidence of thyroid antibodies, for example. On the other hand, there may be minor abnormalities in liver function tests and other signs of liver damage which are not found in true vitiligo. The main histological features seen on liver biopsy include moderate or severe focal fatty change, fibrosis and hepatocellular necrosis. The liver function tests return to normal when exposure to PTBP is discontinued.

Workers exposed to PTBP should be regularly screened with a Wood's lamp to detect those with early vitiligo, and in addition, tests of liver function should be undertaken at periodic intervals.

Prevention

The aim in reducing occupational skin disease is to prevent dangerous substances from coming into contact with the skin. As a preliminary it is necessary to identify those substances which are dangerous and then, wherever possible, enclose the processes in which they are used. When this cannot be done, operators should be given protective clothing, the nature of which will depend on the process and the substance under consideration. Masks and goggles will form part of the protective outfit if appropriate.

Personnel exposed to substances which are liable to produce skin diseases should be told of the potential dangers and informed of the ways in which they can protect themselves. Personal cleanliness is essential and the management should indicate this by seeing to it that standards of factory hygiene are of a high order and by providing good washing facilties and plentiful protective clothing. A factory-based laundry service can sometimes encourage the men to change their overalls more often than they otherwise would.

The use of barrier creams is often advocated. Barrier creams are of three types, (1) simple vanishing creams which fill the pores of the skin with soap thus preventing the entrance of irritants and facilitating their removal by washing, (2) water-repellent creams which prevent water soluble irritants, such as acids and alkalis from coming into contact with the skin, and (3) oil and solvent repellents.

Creams such as these are best provided in dispensers in washrooms since it is essential that they are applied to clean skin otherwise irritants may be trapped under them. It goes without saying that the barrier creams must be non-irritant and this rule ought also to apply to the many proprietary brands of skin cleansers which are available. Unfortunately, this is not always the case, and there are many instances in which dermatitis is caused by skin cleansers. Excessive use of cleansers can lead to drying of the skin and this is so particularly when detergent cleansers are used, the injury often being compounded by virtue of their defatting properties. Of the detergent cleansers, the cationics are more likely to produce skin reactions than the anionics, whilst the non-ionics are the least harmful of the three types available.

The use of solvents to remove materials on the skin must be actively discouraged. Many men working in machine shops are often tempted to remove oil from their skin by this means, and whilst there is no doubt that they achieve this objective, they do so at the risk of causing the skin disease they are trying to avoid. Solvents used in this way are probably the most important cause of dermatitis in machine-room workers, they being tempted into the habit by the unwelcome prospect of the walk to the washroom.

CHAPTER 8/OCCUPATIONAL CANCER

The first recognized association between occupation and malignant disease was made in 1775 by Percivall Pott, a surgeon at St. Bartholomew's Hospital, when he described the occurrence of scrotal cancer in chimney sweeps. Although more tumours of occupational origin have been recognized since Pott's day, both the number of sites at which they occur and the number of undisputed occupational carcinogens is relatively small; there are a great many chemicals which are suspected to be carcinogens on the basis of *in vitro* mutagenicity tests. Some attempts have been made to estimate the proportion of all malignant disease which might be of occupational origin. The results show an extreme variation (from less than 1 per cent to more than half), and are based as much on political or economic considerations as on epidemiology; the true proportion lies towards the lower end of the range and probably does not exceed 5 per cent. Tumours of occupational origin have no pathological features to distinguish them from those which appear to arise spontaneously, nor does their symptomatology differ, but they all share the following characteristics.

1   They tend to appear at an earlier age than tumours which arise in the same sites spontaneously. Because of this, death also occurs at a younger age.

2   They arise as a result of repeated exposure to the putative carcinogen, although the exposure need not be continuous.

3   There is usually a long latent interval between the time of first exposure and the appearance of the tumour. This latent interval is commonly of the order of 20 years or more.

These features, particularly the earlier age of onset, ought to alert doctors to the possibility of an occupational origin for a tumour, but they are of no help in preventing its occurrence. The long latent interval is such that the carcinogenicity of a new material will go unnoticed until many years after its introduction into industrial use unless experiments with animals raise the possibilities of its dangers, or its chemical structure is similar to that of a known carcinogen.

CHEMICAL CARCINOGENS

Experiments which began in the period between the two world wars helped to establish that at least two processes are involved in chemical carcinogenesis, initiation and promotion. Initiation is seen as a process whereby an irreversible potential for malignancy is induced in a target cell; this malignant potential becomes manifest only when the cell is further acted upon by a promotor. Some chemicals act as both initiators and promotors and are referred to as complete carcinogens.

The underlying mechanisms of initiation and promotion are not fully understood, but it is generally considered that the most common event is the induction, by initiators, of mutations in somatic cells. Since not all chemical carcinogens are mutagens, it is clear that some epigenetic phenomena are also involved. For example, chemical carcinogens may affect DNA repair mechanisms leading to an increased proneness to produce faulty genetic material; they may also interact with cellular mediators of genetic expression, alter the cellular response to normal growth control by non-genetic effects or perhaps reduce the efficacy of the immune system.

The majority of initiators are mutagens, however, and initiation, unlike promotion is not dose-dependent. A mutagen changes the structure of the DNA molecule, frequently by changing the sequence of purine or pyrimidine bases in the molecule. The simplest way by which this is achieved is base-pair transformation in which one base is replaced by another. This may be accomplished by chemical modification as, for example, when adenine or cytosine are deaminated to form hypoxanthine or uracil respectively. Alternatively, mutation may be accomplished by the incorporation of an abnormal base analogue into the DNA molecule during replication; the mutagen 5-bromouracil, for example, is an analogue of thymine and will replace it during replication. One or more bases may also be added or deleted from the DNA molecule to produce what is known as a frame-shift mutation. Whatever the mechanism, however, a change in the sequence of bases alters the triplet code and will result in errors in the amino-acid sequence of formed proteins.

Mutagens may also affect whole chromosomes by causing breaks or faulty repair; these effects are similar to the base pair changes but on a grander scale.

Cancer of the skin

Cancer of the scrotum was the first instance of an occupational malignancy to be recognized and Pott's description of the clinical course of the disease has no equal.

> It is a disease which always makes its first attack on, and its first appearance in, the inferior part of the scrotum; where it produces a superficial, painful, ragged, ill-looking sore, with hard and rising edges: the trade call it the sootwart. I never saw it under the age of puberty, which is, I suppose one reason why it is generally taken, both by patient and surgeon, for venereal; and being treated with mercurials, is thereby soon and much exasperated. In no great length of time, it pervades the skin, dartos, and membranes of the scrotum, and seizes the testicle, which it enlarges, hardens, and renders truly and thoroughly distempered; from whence it makes its way up the spermatic process into the abdomen, most frequently indurating and spoiling the inguinal glands: when arrived within the abdomen, it affects some of the viscera, and then very soon becomes painfully destructive.

Since Pott's day occupational skin cancer has been noted to occur at other sites, most usually on exposed skin surfaces. The disease has been recorded in men working with pitch and tar, with arsenic, and in those exposed to mineral oils. In the 1920s and 1930s there was a virtual epidemic in the Lancashire cotton industry which necessitated the introduction of new safety measures and the introduction of oils of low carcinogenicity. More recently men exposed to cutting oils in the engineering industry have been found to be at risk. Agricultural workers are another high-risk group since their outdoor work exposes them to ultra-violet light from the sun. This is not as substantial a hazard in England as in some other more favoured countries. In the early days of radiography, many radiologists unwittingly exposed themselves to high doses of X-rays which produced malignant changes in their skin.

New cases of epitheliomatous ulceration of the skin have to be notified to the Health and Safety Executive and most cases are still due to exposure to pitch and tar, although mineral oil exposure is becoming of increasing importance. Many cases go unnotified, however, because an adequate occupational history is not obtained from the patient.

Men exposed to pitch and tar frequently develop hyperkeratotic lesions which they refer to as warts, on exposed skin. These sometimes fall off, or the men treat themselves with applications of caustic solutions. In the same way, a proportion of men exposed to mineral oils develop folliculitis and hyperkeratotic lesions which in the majority of cases do not become malignant. When malignant change does super-vene, the lesion (or lesions) becomes ulcerated, bleeds and enlarges. Local spread to lymph nodes may be apparent by the time the patient seeks medical advice.

Prevention. Protective clothing and the provision of good washing facilities are essential for men coming into contact with pitch, tar and mineral oil. Unfortunately, most protective clothing is uncomfortable to wear since it is not only impervious to pitch and oil but also to water vapour, so that the workman tends to sweat whilst wearing it. Men at risk should be made aware of the dangers of the substances with which they are working and encouraged to examine their skin regularly and report any suspicious lesions to their own doctor or their works doctor, if there is one. Regular medical inspections may help by detecting growths at an early stage, but these are not yet required by law, except for mule spinners and patent fuel workers, and so the onus is on the works doctor and the men to co-operate in voluntary schemes. Machines on which cutting oils are used are nowadays guarded to prevent splashing and only oils of low carcinogenicity should be used.

Carcinogens in pitch, tar and oil

These are considered to be polycyclic aromatic hydrocarbons, largely concentrated in the fractions with the highest boiling points. A great deal of work has gone into defining mineral oils which have low carcin-ogenicity. Much of the early work was done in Manchester in the wake of the outbreak of skin cancer amongst the mule spinners in the late 1920s. It was then found that the carcinogenic potency of oil could be related to a number of physical properties, the most important of which were the refractive index and the density. More recently, solvent extrac-tion has been used to reduce the carcinogenicity of mineral oils and since the mid-1960s, so-called solvent refined oils have come into general use.

Carcinoma of the bladder

The first cases of occupational bladder cancer were reported in Germany in 1895 as occurring in workers employed in the manufacture of aniline dyes. Thereafter it became common practice to refer to such tumours as aniline tumours although, in fact, aniline was not responsible for their production. Compounds which are responsible for causing bladder tumours are certain aromatic amines used as intermediates in the manufacture of dyes and pharmaceuticals, as antioxidants and accelerators in the rubber industry, and as curing agents for polymerized elastomers in the plastics industry. Some of the more important of these aromatic amines are shown in Figure 8.1.

β-naphthylamine has probably contributed most to the production of bladder cancer in industry and it was withdrawn from use in this country in 1949. The fumes inside gas retort houses may contain β-naphthylamine and this probably accounts for the excess of bladder tumours found in gas workers.

α-naphthylamine in the pure state is usually considered noncarcinogenic but it is difficult to prepare the pure compound for industrial use and it usually contains up to 4 per cent of β-naphthylamine as a contaminant. The difference in activity between the two compounds relates to the position of the NH_2 radical and as a general rule, compounds with a free position para to the NH_2 are noncarcinogenic.

Benzidine was widely used as a laboratory reagent for the detection of occult blood in faeces. Since 1962, however, it has not been used for this purpose in the United Kingdom but in America this use continues. Benzidine is an essential intermediate in the dyestuffs industry. It is not manufactured in this country, however, and can only be imported in the form of its hydrochlorides provided a licence has been obtained and that the compounds contain a minimum of one-third water.

Dimethylbenzidine (o-tolidine) was once used in medical laboratories for occult blood testing but it should now no longer be used as it is carcinogenic in animals and probably in humans also.

Dichlorobenzidine, another analogue of benzidine, is a potent experimental carcinogen but is still used in the dyestuffs industry and for curing polyurethane elastomers. Xenylamine (4-amino diphenyl) is a highly potent carcinogen and is not used in this country.

MOCA (3,3′-dichlor, 4,4′-diamino diphenyl methane)* is used as a hardener for some types of urethane foam rubber. It has been shown to produce lung and liver tumours in experimental animals and to cause haemorrhagic cystitis in men exposed to it. For these reasons its use in industry is kept under close supervision and most manufacturers in this country prefer not to use it. The closely related compound DADPM (4,4′-diamino diphenyl methane) causes liver tumours in rats but it has not been shown to cause bladder cancer. This compound was

*This compound is also known as MbOCA from its alternative chemical name, methylene-bis-o-chloraniline.

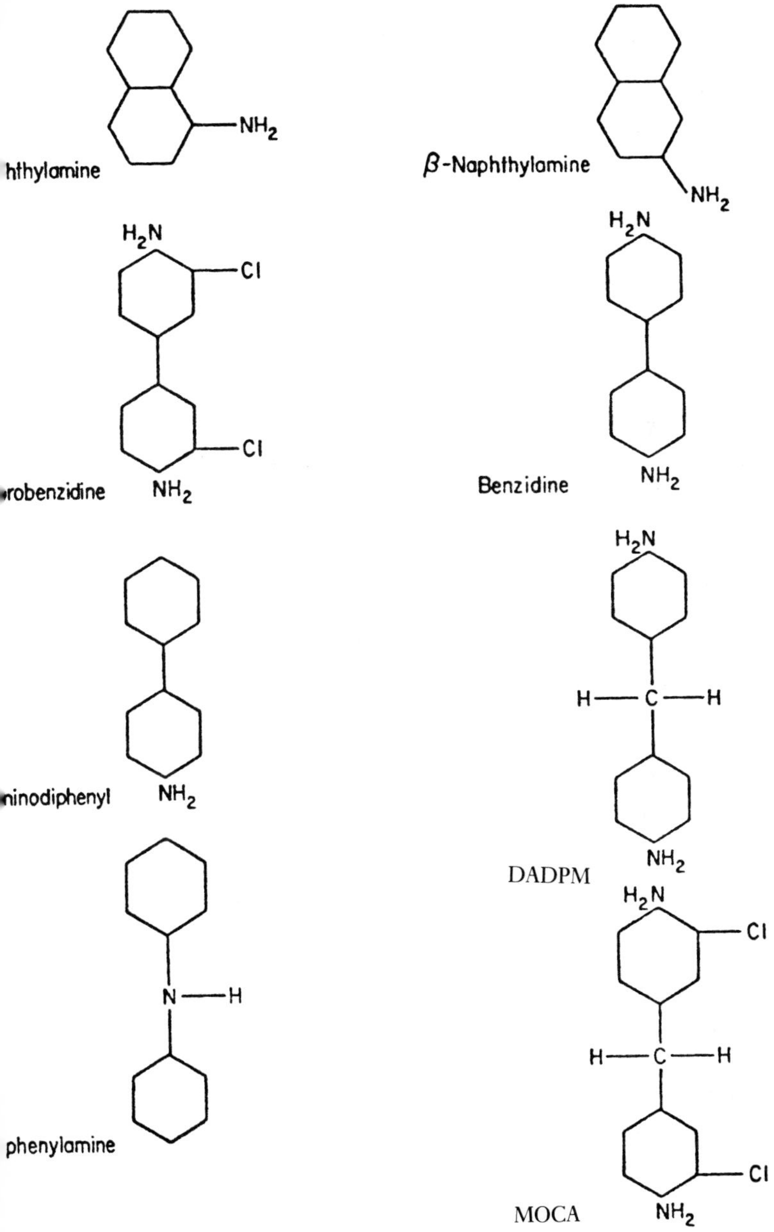

Fig. 8.1. Chemical structure of some important aromatic amines.

responsible for what has become known as the Epping jaundice. A total of 84 people presented with abdominal pain and jaundice and an influenzal-like illness due to eating bread which had become contaminated with DADPM. The lorry in which the sack of flour was transported from the mill to the bakery had previously carried a solution of DADPM, some of which had been spilt on the floor of the lorry. The lorry was not thoroughly cleaned between trips and so the sack containing the flour became impregnated by the residual fluid.

Diphenylamine is used as an intermediary in the dyestuffs industry and in the manufacture of rubber anti-oxidants. There is no evidence that it is carcinogenic in man or animals but it has been found to contain 4-amino diphenyl as an impurity and its use must be closely monitored.

Prevention. The manufacture of compounds which are essential intermediates in the production of important materials and for which no substitute can be found is controlled by a Code of Practice drawn up by the British Association of Chemical Manufacturers. The importation of β-naphthylamine, benzidine, 4-amino diphenyl, 4-nitro diphenyl and their salts, and substances containing them has been prohibited since 1967 except where they are present as a chemical by-product in a concentration not exceeding 1 per cent.

The manufacturing processes in which potentially carcinogenic compounds are used, and the men employed in these processes must obviously be meticulously supervised. The clinical course of the disease is no different from that of the spontaneously occurring variant and early diagnosis affords the best hope of a cure. All those exposed must be warned of the possible dangers in order that they cooperate with monitoring schemes.

Cytological examination of urinary sediment has become an established part of screening procedures for men at risk and should be undertaken at least twice a year, supplemented by cystoscopy when necessary. Malignant cells may be found in the absence of haematuria but the latter sign is always an indication for further investigation.

Other tumours of the renal tract

Tumours of the renal pelvis, the ureter and the urethra have been reported in men exposed to aromatic amines, usually in those who have already had a bladder tumour. The incidence of these tumours is said to be increasing, and relates to the improved survival rate in those with tumours of the bladder. Adenocarcinoma of the kidney is not found to have an increased incidence in workers exposed to aromatic amines. Experimentally these tumours have been induced in rats by lead salts administered either orally or subcutaneously, but no excess of kidney tumours has been shown in industrial lead workers.

Tumours of the liver

Tumours of the liver are occasionally noted in workers exposed to benzidene and they have also been reported in men exposed to arsenical insecticide sprays but these men also had hepatic cirrhosis which has a well-known association with hepatic tumours.

Experimentally, a number of azo dyes and solvents produce liver tumours in animals, but no undue risks appear to be associated with industrial exposure.

Angiosarcoma of the liver has been found in men exposed to VCM. To date less than 30 cases have been reported in the world and the tumour has occurred only in men who have been exposed to very high concentrations, usually those cleaning the reaction vessels. In view of the long latent period it is likely that more cases will appear and a control limit for VCM has recently been introduced.

Cancer of the bronchus

Tumours of the lung were noted to occur amongst the miners of Schneeburg in the Erzgebirge. Later the uranium miners in Joachimstal, on the other side of the Erzgebirge, were also found to be subject to a high risk of developing bronchial tumours. The mines were worked successively for silver, nickel, and uranium and provided the ore from which the Curies isolated radium. There was a very high level of radioactivity in both mines and many years later, when the ventilation had been substantially improved, the average concentration of radon in the air was 3×10^{-9} curies/litre. Radon decays to form a series of daughter products with the emission of α-particles. There is no doubt that the α-particles are the carcinogenic agent and they produce an undifferentiated carcinoma which arises from the bronchial epithelium. It has been suggested that when conditions were at their worst, the miners in the Schneeburg and Joachimstal mines were receiving doses of 100,000 rads of α-particles to the lungs.

The increased risk of lung cancer experienced by uranium miners in other areas of the world is also due to exposure to radon.

Uranium miners, however, are by no means alone in their occupational exposure to radon since the gas is found in almost all metaliferrous mines, sometimes in concentrations which are in excess of the limits laid down by the atomic energy industry for their own workers.

Nickel

Tumours of the lung were a risk to those employed refining nickel from its ores by the Mond process, but this risk now seems to have disappeared, although it is still experienced by those refining nickel by electrolytic processes. Men who ran the greatest risk in the Mond process were those engaged in calcining the ore or in extracting the ore with sulphuric acid which contained large amounts of arsenic. In 1920–4 an acid which was virtually free of arsenic was substituted and thereafter, the risk declined. This has led to speculation that the arsenic was responsible for the disease, but not all authorities agree. Nickel in powdered form has been shown to be carcinogenic to animals and the reduction in airborne dust due to improvements in the process is a more likely reason for the decline.

Carcinoma of the nasal passages has also been attributed to exposure to nickel, but as with lung cancer, the risk appears to have diminished in recent years. Adeno-carcinoma of the nose and air sinuses, however, is still a risk for men in the furniture industry exposed to wood dust and to a lesser extent, for men using leather in the shoemaking industry.

Chromates

Workers manufacturing chromates from chrome ores have been shown to have a higher than expected incidence of lung tumours, mono-chromate ores seeming to represent the greatest hazard. Exposure to dichromates frequently give rise to ulcers of the skin and the nasal septum but these do not undergo malignant change.

Asbestos

There is no doubt that prolonged exposure to asbestos may lead to the development of bronchial carcinoma and about half of those who develop asbestosis die from lung cancer; it is debatable whether lung cancer develops in an asbestos worker in the absence of asbestosis. Not only the degree of exposure but also the type of exposure is important, however. Thus, the risk of developing lung cancer is much greater in those who have been engaged in the manufacture of asbestos products than in those who have worked in mining or milling processes. This difference is probably due to the fact that a higher proportion of sub-microscopic fibres is produced during textile manufacture than during mining and milling. Cigarette smoking considerably enhances the risk of lung cancer in those exposed to asbestos.

Gas-workers

Men who have worked in retort houses in gas works experience a higher risk than normal of developing cancer of the bronchus. The tarry material which is produced during the process of distillation of coal to make coal gas contains a large number of polycyclic aromatic hydro-carbons which are found also in the generated fumes. This fume contains benzo (a) pyrene and in the horizontal retort houses very high concentrations ($> 200\mu gm^{-3}$) were recorded above the retorts. Apart from this special case, there are no differences in the concentrations of benzo (a) pyrene in horizontal retort houses and vertical retort houses, although there is an increased risk of lung cancer in the horizontal as opposed to the vertical retort houses. It is not clear how far this difference can be accounted for in terms of the experience of the men who worked in the most polluted areas.

Haematite

The iron ore miners in West Cumberland who work underground experience an occupational risk of lung cancer about 70 per cent greater than normal. Miners working on the surface do not have the same risk. Also in France, iron ore miners have been found to have a similar lung cancer risk. As mentioned earlier, the risk arises because of exposure to radon. In the Cumberland mines, the average radon concentration in the air is 100 Ci/l.

Mesothelioma

This rare tumour affecting principally the pleura, but also the peri-toneum, is particularly a hazard of exposure to crocidolite but other forms of asbestos will, with the exception of antophyllite, produce the disease. Crocidolite from the north-west Cape Province is far more dangerous in this respect than crocidolite from the Transvaal. The exposure need not be prolonged and nonoccupational cases are known in persons living in the neighbourhood of asbestos factories or mines.

The main symptom is dyspnoea which rapidly increases in severity and may be accomanied by cough, haemoptysis and chest pain. A chest X-ray will demonstrate massive thickening of the pleura with pleural effusion and perhaps signs of lung collapse. Straw-coloured pleural fluid, often blood-stained, can be aspirated from the chest and malignant cells will be found on cytological examination. Abdominal tumours give rise to ascites with a bloody exudate containing malignant cells.

The tumour is a dense white growth which may spread to the whole of the lung and cause collapse. Ultimately the whole pleural cavity becomes obliterated. The pericardium may become affected and the mediastium becomes progressively widened by tumour growth. Peritoneal tumours sometimes involve all the abdominal organs but more usually the growth is unevenly distributed. Metastatic spread is not common but in some cases there is a generalized lymphadenopathy and subcutaneous nodules may be found over the neck and chest. Rarely nodules are found on the tongue. The diagnoses should be confirmed by pleural biopsy but no treatment is sufficient to prevent the fatal outcome of the disease and this takes months rather than years.

Leukaemia

Ionizing radiation

Ionizing radiation is well known to produce leukaemia in experimental animals and in man. The evidence for the latter association has come from the increased rates which were formerly shown in radiologists and others working in diagnostic X-ray units, in patients irradiated for ankylosing spondylitis and in survivors of the atomic bomb explosions in Hiroshima and Nagasaki. The relationship between the mean dose of radiation to the spinal marrow and the age-standardized incidence of leukaemia in patients with ankylosing spondylitis is shown in Table 8.1. It should be noted that the doses to which these patients were exposed are much higher than those which could be encountered by patients undergoing diagnostic radiology or by persons who are exposed to radiation either in hospitals or in industry during the course of their occupation. Nevertheless, ionizing radiation is becoming increasingly used in both situations and there is no room for anything but the most stringent control (see Chapter 9).

Benzene

Exposure to benzene has occasionally been found to result in the production of leukaemia, frequently superimposed as a terminal event on aplastic anaemia. The myeloid types are the most common, but all other varieties have been recorded from time to time.

Table 8.1. Standardized incidence rates for leukaemia in men with ankylosing spondylitis after different doses of irradiation to the spinal marrow*

Mean dose, rads	0	250	750	1250	1750	2500
Standardized incidence rate/ 10,000 men/year	0.49	1.98	4.66	7.21	13.44	72.16

*From Court-Brown W.M. and Doll R., *Medical Research Council Special Report* Series No. 295, HMSO, 1957.

Other volatile solvents such as toluene and xylene have sometimes been incriminated as causing leukaemia, but as used industrially they often contain large amounts of benzene as an impurity. There is no evidence that in the pure state they are capable of inducing malignant changes in the marrow.

Osteosarcoma

Radium salts were first used in industry in the manufacture of luminous paint which was then applied to watch and clock faces with brushes. The girls employed in this work kept the point on their brushes by licking them, and in this way they swallowed considerable quantities of the radioactive paint. A high proportion of the girls subsequently developed anaemia and necrosis of the jaw, but in addition some also developed osteosarcomata. This process now takes place under carefully controlled conditions.

TESTING CHEMICALS FOR CARCINOGENICITY

In many countries manufacturers are not permitted to introduce new chemicals into use unless they have undergone carcinogenicity tests. The testing schedules are laid down by the regulating authorities in the countries concerned and vary one from another. In general, however, the schedule requires both *in vitro* and *in vivo* tests.

In vitro *tests:* Because they are relatively quick and cheap, there has been a great deal of effort in recent years to develop reliable *in vitro* tests of carcinogenicity. Many are available but the one which is still in most common use is the Ames' test which actually determines the ability of chemicals to induce a specific mutation in bacteria. Another frequently used test, technically more difficult than the Ames' test, measures the ability of chemical compounds to induce transformations in cell cultures. It is also a test of mutagenicity but this is accepted as satisfactory since the majority of chemical carcinogens are also mutagens. There is no absolute certainty, however, that the converse is true, that is, that all mutagens are also carcinogens. Nevertheless, short term tests may be used to screen chemicals in the first instance and *in vivo* tests are usually required only if at least two *in vitro* tests give positive results.

The Ames' test relies on the ability of chemicals to induce a mutation in a histidine requiring strain of *Salmonella typhimurium.* To conduct the test, the chemical is mixed with the bacteria and an enzyme rich rat liver fraction. It is invariably the case that the active carcinogens (or mutagens) are metabolites of the parent compound and the liver fraction is thus essential to ensure that this transformation takes place. The mixture is then plated out onto nutrient agar which lacks histidine and incubated for 3 days. After this, the number of revertant colonies, that is those which have derived from a mutant not requiring histidine, is counted. The background reversion rate is low, of the order of 10 or less colonies whereas in the presence of a mutagen the count may be as high as 10^4 per plate.

In vivo *tests:* With *in vivo* tests, a compound may be tested for carcinogenicity rather than for mutagenicity. Various protocols exist for carrying out these tests, but all are time consuming and expensive. One which is commonly used is that proposed by the National Cancer Institutes of America. The dose to be used in the study is determined by a preliminary subacute study carried out on rats and mice of both sexes. The animals are tested in groups of 5 and 6 dose levels are administered for 42 weeks followed by a 2-week observation period. From these experiments the maximum tolerated dose (MTD) is determined and for the main study, animals are given a high (MTD) or a low (0.5 MTD) oral dose of the chemical for 5 days a week for 78 weeks. This period is followed by further observation, the extent of which is variable but may be until 80 per cent of the animals have died. The animals which have survived until the end of the experiment are then sacrificed and a full pathological examination is carried out and a histological examination is made of any tumours present; those animals which have died before the end of the experiment will already have been treated likewise. The prevalence of tumours in the experimental animals and in control animals is then determined.

Chemicals which are shown unequivocally to be carcinogenic or mutagenic must clearly be treated with the utmost caution and not introduced into use unless there are over-riding reasons for doing so and there is no suitable alternative. Positive results in *in vivo* or *in vitro* tests, however, must not necessarily lead to the conclusion that the chemicals in question are human carcinogens. With a number of chemicals the dose which is needed to produce tumours in animals is far in excess of that which would be encountered in industrial use and the mode of administration is often different; in many test schedules an oral dose is given whereas in industry the major route of entry is by inhalation or, to a lesser degree, through the skin. Thus, trichloroethylene has been found to induce hepatic tumours in mice when given in massive oral doses but there is no evidence that it is carcinogenic in man. It should also be remembered that chemical carcinogens do not propduce the same effects in all species. For example, tar has little carcinogenic effect on the skin of rats or dogs whereas in mice and rabbits tumours are produced with ease. Conversely, mice and rabbits are relatively unresponsive to β-naphthylamine which produces bladder tumours in dogs. A recent report that exposure to formaldehyde produced tumours of the nasal sinuses in rats set in train a series of human epidemiological studies, none of which produced positive results. The cause of this particular discrepancy seems to lie in the anatomy of the rat's nose; it has extremely large ethmoids with a large surface area for absorption and it is thus prone to the effects of substances which are mucosal irritants.

Despite these caveats it is obviously prudent to treat mutagenic substances with circumspection taking care to tread the narrow line between alarmism and indifference. Moreover, it must also be remembered that materials which are not animal carcinogens may nevertheless be carcinogenic to man and only long usage will give a definite answer.

'NONSPECIFIC' CANCER

Some occupations involve exposure to specific carcinogenic hazards and the site of the disease is characteristic for the occupation; bladder in rubber workers, mesothelioma in asbestos workers, skin in oil workers and so on. Certain other occupations, however, appear to have an excess risk of developing tumours in various sites, even though, in most cases there is no well-recognized specific hazard.

In Table 8.2 a list of these occupations and the tumour sites is shown. The data have been taken from the Occupational Mortality Tables of the Registrar General and to avoid the social class bias discussed in Chapter 1, only those occupations in which there is an excess in the men but not their wives (as indicated by a significant t-value) are shown.

There is only one case in which it is possible to suggest a specific carcinogenic hazard and that is for the excess of bladder carcinoma in gas, coke and chemical workers where exposure to aromatic amines is the probable carcinogenic risk. Otherwise it is difficult to see the connection between the occupation and the apparent enhanced risk of malignancy. In all probability, however, there are many carcinogens, or groups of carcinogens acting in concert, which have not been identified, and this is a fertile region for epidemiological exploration.

Table 8.2. Malignant causes of death, by occupation, with high t-values in men but not their wives

Site of cancer	Occupation
Mouth	Textile workers
Oesophagus	Food, drink and tobacco workers
Stomach	Gas, coke and chemical workers
	Furnace, forge, foundry, rolling mill workers
	Painters and decorators
Rectum	Furnace, forge, foundry, rolling mill workers
Pancreas	Clothing workers
Larynx, lung, bronchus and trachea	Food, drink and tobacco workers
	Glass and ceramic makers
	Furnace, forge, foundry, rolling mill workers
	Electrical and electronic workers
	Construction workers
	Painters and decorators
	Warehousemen, storekeepers, packers, bottlers
Kidney	Electrical and electronic workers
Bladder and other urinary organs	Gas, coke and chemical makers
	Transport and communication workers
Bone	Furnace, forge, foundry, rolling mill workers

From the Registrar General's *Occupational Mortality Tables*, HMSO, 1971.

CHAPTER 9/PHYSICAL HAZARDS

DECOMPRESSION SICKNESS

This syndrome can occur in three groups of persons.

1 Those working in compressed air who are too rapidly decompressed,

2 Divers who surface too rapidly from depths greater than about 33 feet (10 metres),

3 Crew or paratroopers in aircraft who ascend too rapidly from sea level to heights of greater than 18,000 feet (5487 metres).

In the first category the syndrome is sometimes called caisson disease, after the apparatus which is used when underwater excavation is being carried out during the course of constructing piers, bridges, etc. The caisson is an iron or concrete tube open at the bottom, which is weighted and driven into the mud or sand below water. The men working in the caisson descend through a series of airtight chambers in which the atmospheric pressure is successively raised. It is the high atmospheric pressure in the final working chamber which prevents it from being flooded. The usual maximum working pressures in compressed air work in building or in civil engineering is 4.5 kg/cm^3 (441.2 × 10^3 Pa) and generally much less. When the worker ascends back to the surface, the air pressure is reduced to atmospheric as he passes through successive chambers.

The manifestations of decompression sickness are due to the formation of nitrogen bubbles in the body fluids and in the tissues. Bubbles of nitrogen large enough to cause symptoms form when the partial pressure of nitrogen in the tissues rapidly becomes twice as great as its partial pressure in the atmosphere.

The symptoms produced depend upon the site in which the bubbles are formed whilst the size and rate of growth of the bubbles determines the severity of the symptoms.

Symptoms: The acute symptoms of decompression sickness are usually divided into two types (see Table 9.1); some chronic symptoms also occur.

Table 9.1. Symptoms in different types of decompression sickness

Type I	Mild or severe limb pain
	Skin mottling or skin irritation
Type II	Paralysis or weakness of the limbs
	Tingling or numbness in the limbs
	Vertigo
	Headache
	Dyspnoea
	Fits or convulsions
	Chest pain
	Hypotension
	Coma
Chronic	Aseptic necrosis of the bones
	Neurological or psychological symptoms

Type I: The main symptom is acute pain in the limbs usually in the joints, sometimes preceded by numbness; the pain may come on at any time during the 12 hours following decompression. The affected part is often held in a semi-flexed position from which it is difficult to move, hence this condition is known amongst divers as the bends. Skin mottling and itching may occur with or without joint pain.

Type II: Type II symptoms are much more serious than Type I but are seen much more rarely. The most striking are paralysis of one or more limbs which may be accompanied by vertigo, nausea or vomiting. If nitrogen bubbles occur in the pulmonary vasculature the worker experiences a sensation of burning retrosternal distress with a cough. This may be at first relieved by shallow breathing but after a while the coughing becomes paroxysmal and uncontrollable. These symptoms are referred to as the chokes. In the most serious cases the patient may pass into a coma and die unless immediate treatment is given. Post-decompression shock with haemoconcentration is another serious complication.

Aseptic necrosis

Aseptic necrosis of bone is thought to result from infarcts brought about by nitrogen emboli lodging in the nutrient arteries (Fig. 9.1). The changes are often symmetrical but the condition is only serious or disabling if the articular surfaces of the humerus or femur are affected. About a quarter of all compressed air workers have aseptic necrosis but only 3 per cent are disabled. By contrast, aseptic necrosis is seen in only about 5 per cent of deep sea divers and only about 0.2 per cent are disabled.

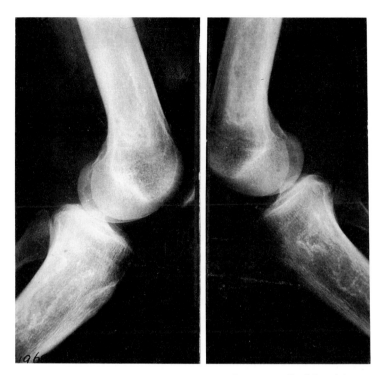

Fig. 9.1. Radiographs showing aseptic necrosis in the bones around both knee joints in a naval diver.

Prevention and treatment: In most cases decompression work is carried out in accordance with a statutory set of tables many of which have been based on the 1958 British tables which owed much to the work of Haldane. In the UK these tables have now been superseded by the Blackpool Decompression Tables which are published in the Medical Code of Practice for Work in Compressed Air.

Men who are to work at reduced atmospheres should be carefully selected, weeding out the fat, the alcoholic and those with pre-existing cardiovascular or pulmonary disease. Men over 35 years of age are also best not newly recruited. A radiographic examination of the chest and the major joints should be carried out and the major joints should be

X-rayed every 2 years. Anyone who has had Type II symptoms must not be allowed to work in decompressed conditions again unless there are the most overwhelming reasons for him to do so.

The symptoms of decompression sickness are relieved by recompressing the patient and reducing the pressure in accordance with a protocol laid down in a set of tables; the one contained in the US Navy Diving Manual is frequently used.

Other effects of diving or increased atmospheric pressure

Divers are at risk from several other hazards which may or may not be due to increased atmospheric pressure. The risk of drowning is ever-present and this is far and away the most common cause of death in divers. At great depths there is the danger from cold and some provision must be made to maintain the normal body temperature. Anyone who dives into water—whether using breathing apparatus or not—may develop a spontaneous pneumothorax if he surfaces too rapidly; he also runs the risk of being attacked by other creatures in the sea.

When the pressure on a diver exceeds 4 atmospheres (equal to about 100 feet or 30 metres of water) a diver breathing air may suffer from nitrogen narcosis. Judgement, thought and movement all become impaired and if the diver does not surface, he may become unconscious. The symptoms rapidly clear when the diver returns to normal pressure. Substituting helium for nitrogen in a breathing apparatus prevents the onset of symptoms.

Adverse effects are also noted from exposure to high partial pressures of oxygen. Divers breathing pure oxygen are at risk in depths greater than 25 feet (7½ metres) and those breathing helium/oxygen mixtures are at some risk at very great depths (greater than 500 feet or 150 metres) and a vague feeling of discomfort may precede more serious symptoms, but convulsions and coma can occur with little warning.

All divers using oxygen apparatus should be able to recognize the symptoms of oxygen narcosis and come to the surface as soon as they notice them. The only treatment required is to breathe fresh air.

Patients in hyperbaric chambers and their attendants should also be on their guard against oxygen poisoning.

HEAT

So-called heat cramps may be a symptom amongst forge and foundry workers, metal casters, iron and glass workers, and miners, as well as those who work out of doors in hot climates. They may also occur as the result of heat generated by microwave radiation. The incidence of the disease shows seasonal variations, well over three-quarters of the cases occurring during the summer months.

The symptoms usually occur during the second half of the shift and those affected are generally of poor physique. Sometimes there are prodromal symptoms such as headache and dizziness, but characteristically there is a sudden onset of severe cramping pain in the muscles being used at the time. Most often the attack begins in the calves and spreads to the muscles of the upper limbs and abdomen. The pains are of an intermittent nature, occurring with increasing severity every few minutes. Albuminuria is frequently found but there are no other abnormal signs.

The condition is, in effect, a form of water intoxication, brought about because the workman drinks a lot of water in response to the sweating experienced in the hot environment, which, in turn, leads to a decrease in the plasma osmolality. Treatment with a drink containing sodium chloride is all that is required in the way of treatment. In factories where it is impossible to eliminate the heat hazard entirely, a stock of tablets from which such drinks can be made should be kept for use by the men at work. If they drink this salt solution regularly, the symptoms do not appear.

Men who work regularly in a hot environment gradually become acclimatized and it is found that they conserve sodium and chloride so that the concentration of these ions in the sweat falls. This phenomenon explains why heat cramps are not more common.

Heat exhaustion and heat stroke

Heat exhaustion is associated with a depletion of both salt and water. The concentration of the body fluids is not altered greatly but there is a dimunition in blood volume which accounts for the symptoms. Over a period of a few days the patient complains of weakness, fatigue and headache, with perhaps anorexia and vomiting. If the vomiting is persistent, circulatory collapse may follow. Generally the patient is incapacitated before this stage is reached and the disease is rarely fatal.

When seen by the doctor, the patient will have signs of peripheral circulatory failure with pallor, hypotension and profuse sweating. There is generally little elevation of the body temperature.

Treatment consists of removing the patient to a cool place, rest in bed and replacement of salt and water, which can be achieved in the majority of cases by the oral route. If the patient is severely ill, recourse to intravenous replacement will be necessary.

In heat stroke, the symptoms are due to a defect in thermoregulation producing a positive heat balance. The onset is abrupt. The patient falls unconscious and is found to have a temperature of at least 40.6°C. Management consists of rapid cooling by whatever means possible and the aim must be to reduce the temperature to 40°C within 1 hour, thus minimizing the danger of damage to the central nervous system.

Treatment may be required for as long as a week before sweating returns and the patient is able to regulate his temperature unaided.

Neither of these conditions is likely to be encountered with any frequency in this country.

OCCUPATIONAL CATARACTS

Most cases of occupational cataracts are the late result of penetrating injuries to the eye, although in the past heat-induced cataracts were the most common variety. Cataracts may also be a sequelae of exposure to ionizing radiation and may follow an electric shock.

Traumatic cataracts

These follow penetrating injuries to the eye in which the lens capsule is ruptured, although they do sometimes form following a simple contusion to the eye with no penetration.

The hazard is particularly great where men are using explosives or working on lathes and presses, where small pieces of metal may fly into the eye. Protective goggles should be worn by all men at risk but this ideal is seldom achieved.

Heat cataracts

In the early part of the century this form of cataract was common amongst glass-blowers and it was subsequently reported in other workers exposed to radiant energy, most notably chain-makers and furnacemen. The cataract was often unilateral, forming in the eye closest to the source of the heat. It has since become established that X-irradiation of the eye can produce a cataract, the minimum dose for this effect being about 500 rad. Fast neutrons are particularly hazardous in cataract production.

In all cases of radiation cataract the lens changes began in the posterior pole of the lens immediately under the posterior capsule. The opacity was often disc-shaped and had a golden colour when viewed through a slit lamp. In time the opacity spread to involve the remainder of the posterior cortex. The anterior cortex also became involved in the disease process and ultimately the cataract became indistinguishable from the ordinary senile form. The pathognomonic change of a radiation-induced cataract was said to be the exfoliation of the zonula lamella of the anterior capsule. This lamella peeled off in sheets and it was said that in the absence of this change it was difficult to blame an occupational exposure for the production of the posterior cataract.

Heat cataract is seldom met with nowadays. Bottles are usually made mechanically so that one of the most potent sources of hazard has been removed through an advance in technology. Where exposure to heat is unavoidable, workers are protected by wearing goggles made from glass containing metallic oxides which cut off heat radiation but transmit light. Standards for such goggles are laid down by the British Standards Institute.

Electric shock

Rarely, cataract formation has been noted following electric shock. The cataract may be present only on the side on which electrical contact was made or it may be bilateral. There is usually a delay of a year or so before it begins to form, but thereafter it often matures rapidly. Spontaneous regression sometimes occurs within a few weeks of the onset of the lens changes.

Microwave radiation

There have been some reports of cataract formation in workers exposed to relatively high intensity microwave radiation, usually above $100\,\mathrm{mW/cm^2}$, but the association is controversial. It is less readily accepted as proven in the countries of western Europe than in the east principally because, in none of the published reports, has it been possible unequivocally to rule out other causes for the cataracts.

Treatment: The treatment of cataract is the same regardless of the means of formation. The affected lens is removed and the sight defect corrected by suitable spectacles.

MINER'S NYSTAGMUS

This condition is thought to result from poor lighting conditions underground. The relative absence of rods at the macula causes a defect in fixation which is often symptomless. Where there are symptoms they are, in addition to nystagmus, those of vertigo, photophobia, headache, insomnia and blepharospasm. The vertigo may be so severe as to be disabling but in cases where this is so, there appears to be a considerable functional overlay. Defective vision is sometimes reported, but there is no retinal lesion to account for it.

Improvements in lighting underground, including the provision of reflecting surfaces have done much to minimize the condition. Patients who develop symptoms should be reassured that there will be no permanent loss of vision but it may be necessary, nevertheless, to find alternative work for those who are severely affected.

IONIZING RADIATION

The number of radiation sources has increased spectacularly during the last 2 or 3 decades as they find ever wider application both in industry and in hospital practice.

Ionizing radiation can be divided into two main groups; electromagnetic radiations, such as X-rays and γ-rays and corpuscular radiations such as α-particles, β-particles (electrons), protons and neutrons. Unlike the first three particles, neutrons carry no electric charge.

When X-rays or γ-rays are absorbed, high-energy electrons are produced in the irradiated tissue and it is these β-particles which are the effective ionizing agents, being capable of breaking chemical bonds to release positively and negatively charged ions. The radioactive particles are capable of ionization with no intermediary, but for all practical purposes there is no distinction between the biological effects of the different groups.

Definitions

Different units are used to define absorption, dose equivalence and radioactivity.

Absorption is measured in grays (Gy); 1 Gy is defined as an energy absorption of 1 joule per kilogram. It can be applied to all sources of radiation but since not all sources produce equivalent effects in the tissues it is customary to introduce a modifying factor which allows for this variation. The value of the modifying factor, which is sometimes known as the Relative Biological Effectiveness (RBE) is 1 for gamma rays, X-rays and β-particles whereas for α-particles, fast neutrons and protons it is 10. The product of the RBE and the absorbed dose provides the dose equivalent in sieverts (Sv).

The dose equivalent provides an index of the risk of harm following exposure to radiation. Not all the tissues are equally at risk from radiation, however, and to account for this, a series of risk weighting factors has been recommended as shown in Table 9.2.

Table 9.2. Risk weighting factors for ionizing radiation

Tissue or organ	Factor
Gonads	0.25
Breast	0.15
Red bone marrow	0.12
Lung	0.12
Thyroid	0.03
Bone surfaces	0.03
Remainder	0.03

If a single tissue is irradiated the dose can be converted to a dose equivalent for the whole body by applying the appropriate weighting factor. If, as is more common, several tissues are involved, then the weighting factors can be applied to each and the sum of the products is the dose equivalent to the whole body which would yield the same overall risk. The sum of the weighted dose equivalents is known as the effective dose equivalent and is also expressed in sieverts.

Radioactivity is measured in becquerels (Bq), 1 Bq being equivalent to the quantity of radioactive material in which there is one disintegration per second.

Effects of radiation

Acute radiation syndrome: Doses of whole body irradiation of the order of 5–20 Gy delivered over a short period of time results in severe tissue destruction and death within a week. With lower doses, say about 1–5 Gy the patient will survive long enough to develop the acute radiation syndrome, although this will seldom be of much comfort to him. In the typical case, four more or less distinct stages can be distinguished. There is first a short latent period of a few hours during which no ill effects are observed. The second stage is heralded in by nausea and vomiting which passes off within about 24 hours to be followed by a period of minor symptoms including malaise, anorexia, diarrhoea, thirst and lassitude. These persist for a few days and then the patient enters the third stage of comparative well-being although anorexia and malaise may persist and there may be a low-grade fever. After about 3 weeks the patient enters the final stage. If the dose has exceeded 2 Gy a sudden loss of hair may sometimes precede the other symptoms by a few days. Total loss of body hair is a bad prognostic sign since this generally indicates a whole body exposure of at least 5 Gy. Symptoms of this final stage include increasing malaise with pains in the throat and mouth, both of which become inflamed, oedematous and ulcerated. Blood examination at this time reveals profound thrombocytopaenia and leucopaenia which give rise to purpuric haemorrhages, epistaxis and bloody diarrhoea. The bleeding, or an overwhelming infection, is likely to kill the patient, and even if it does not, then the severe damage sustained by the gastro-intestinal tract will produce chronic diarrhoea and a more gradual demise.

The time scale described above may, in very severe cases, be considerably shortened or it may be considerably delayed. If part of the body is shielded from the radiation, then recovery is greatly assisted, generally by a much greater amount than would be expected.

If the patient is to recover, he must survive long enough to allow the cells of his bone marrow and his gastric and intestinal mucosa to recover and repair the damage. During this time, blood transfusions, platelet transfusions, intravenous feeding and prompt antibiotic therapy will be required to support him.

Chronic effects of radiation

Conditions which produce the acute radiation syndrome are, fortunately, very rare, although minor accidents are not uncommon. In industry, serious radiation hazards are likely to be encountered only in critical accidents in establishments handling fissile materials. Chronic effects from radiation of which carcinogenesis, leukaemogenesis and genetic disturbance are the most important, are potentially a greater hazard. Cataract formation is discussed elsewhere (p. 168).

Carcinogenesis

Many different types of tumour have been found to have increased frequency in irradiated populations. These include tumours of the skin in those radiologists who were working when X-rays had just been introduced into medical practice, carcinoma of the lung in miners in Schneeburg and Joachimstal, thyroid carcinoma in patients given irradiation to the neck in childhood for thymic enlargement, tumours of the reticuloendothelial system in patients given Thorotrast* and osteosarcomas in the girls painting luminous watches with radium and other radioactive elements. The survivors of the two nuclear bomb explosions in Japan have developed a number of different types of tumour in addition to having shown an earlier increased incidence of leukaemia. Patients who had received irradiation therapy for ankylosing spondylitis were also found to be more at risk from leukaemia.

An attempt has been made to quantify the increased risk of cancer on the basis of a linear dose/response relationship. The International Commission on Radiological Protection has estimated the number of cases of cancer likely to occur in a population of a million persons each exposed to 0.01 Gy (Table 9.3). Their estimates should not be taken to be precise, however, but rather as showing a trend. The increased incidence of leukaemia found to result from irradiation given for the treatment of ankylosing spondylitis is shown in Table 8.1).

Table 9.3. Estimated risk of cancer from exposure to 0.01 Gy[1]

Type of cancer	Estimated no. of cases per 10^6 persons exposed[2]
Fatal neoplasms:	
Leukaemia[3]	20
Others	20
Thyroid carcinoma[4]	10–20

[1] A linear dose-response relationship is assumed. Since the evidence is based on irradiation by X-rays or γ-rays, the absorbed dose is approximately equal to 1 mSv

[2] Effects would be experienced over 10–20 years.

[3] Risk may be enhanced by a factor of 2–10 if the fetus is exposed.

[4] Estimated refers to exposure in childhood. Unlike other types of cancer for which estimates are given, incidence is not equivalent to mortality.

Based on data from International Commission on Radiological Protection, *The Evaluation of Risks from Radiation*, Pergamon Press, 1966.

*Thorotrast is a collodial suspension of thorium dioxide formerly used as a contrast medium.

Genetic effects

It is generally assumed that irradiation during pregnancy carries a risk to the developing fetus and may cause childhood leukaemia. Diagnostic X-rays to the abdomen are discouraged in pregnant women and in other women should be restricted to the 10 days following the onset of menstruation.

Radiation protection

The philosophy underlying all schemes of radiation protection is that exposure to any amount of ionizing radiation carries some risk of harm. Therefore no exposure is permissible unless there is a benefit associated with the exposure. The benefit may not necessarily be received by the person exposed, but may be a benefit to society as a whole. The dose which an exposed person, or society as a whole, receives must, therefore be kept as low as possible taking into account all the social and economic costs. There are recommended maximum dose limits for both the general public and for radiation workers (see Table 9.4); in practice in the UK, received doses are much lower than those shown in the Table 9.4; the average annual effective dose for radiation workers is 4 mSv whilst for the general public the average effective dose from occupational sources is 9 μSv per year and approximately 530 μSv per year from all sources.

Table 9.4. Dose limits (mSv per year) for radiation workers and members of the general public

	Worker	General public
Effective dose equivalent	50	5
Dose equivalent to single organ or tissue	500	50
Dose equivalent to the eye	300	30

The doses which radiation workers in the UK receive are routinely monitored by the National Radiation Protection Board and a national register of such workers has been established in which lifetime dose and cause of death are recorded. As the data accumulate, it should be possible to determine whether the causes of death differ as between radiation workers and a comparable group not exposed to radiation, and between groups of radiation workers with different lifetime dose levels.

Radioactive elements

A large number of radioactive elements are used in industry, in universities and other research establishments and in hospitals for diagnostic purposes. The principles governing the use of radionuclides are the same as for the use of any other source of ionizing radiation; when being administered to volunteers (and patients count as volunteers) it is now a legal requirement throughout the countries of the European Community that prior authorization must be obtained. This authorization must take into account the training and experience of the practitioner, the facilities which he has at his disposal and the types and amount of radionuclides to be used. Radionuclides are classified according to their toxicity per unit activity and use of the most toxic is very restricted. It goes without saying, that patients and volunteers should be properly advised of the procedure and the degree of risk attached to the procedure so that their consent is truly informed.

When using radionuclides, precautions must be taken not only to avoid exposure to the radiation but also to prevent the unsealed sources from coming into contact with the skin or being taken into the body accidentally. Great care must be given to the design of units in which radionuclides are to be handled, and to the disposal of all waste materials. Sealed sources generally present no problems and they can safely be stored until they have decayed to a low activity or are collected by an approved disposal service. The doses used in experiments are low and most waste will be only minimally contaminated and items such as swabs or paper towels can generally be disposed of normally or held for a time until they have decayed to safe levels. Some items may require special laundering. The urine from patients receiving radio-iodine therapy for thyroid carcinoma may be sufficiently radioactive to require retainment with appropriate shielding until the activity has decayed to safe levels, but otherwise, the excreta from subjects who have been administered radionuclides do not present a hazard. Gaseous wastes may arise from radium stores or fume cupboards or from incinerator stacks. Any point of release must be sited so that the gas is rapidly diluted and unable to re-enter the building from which it was emitted.

The activity of radionuclides used for experimental or industrial work is usually so low that it presents no serious hazard provided that normal work practices are adhered to. The supervision of the use of radionuclides should be in the hands of an expert Radiation Protection Officer who would be an ex officio member of any works safety committee. Hospital workers should be carefully instructed in the safe way to handle excreta or vomit from patients treated with radionuclides; there is no danger from implanted sources. Because the degree of exposure is low, it is not necessary to undertake any form of routine monitoring of workers handling radioactive elements; some special investigations may be required if they suffer accidental contamination.

NON-IONIZING RADIATION

Electro-magnetic radiations with a wavelength greater than 10 nm are incapable of ionizing biological important atoms or molecules because their energy (10 eV) is not sufficiently great and so it is conventionally referred to as non-ionizing. The following categories of non-ionizing radiation are of importance in occupational health practice, ultra-violet (UV), infra-red (IR) and microwave and radiofrequency (MW/RF); lasers will also be considered here.

Ultra-violet radiation

It is usual to categorize UV radiation into two types on the basis of their harmful potential. UVA occurs in the wavelength 315–400 nm and has relatively little biological effect beyond causing mild erythema and pigmentation. UVB, wavelength 280–315 nm, produces much more serious effects on the skin and on the eyes. It causes marked erythema with a peak effect at 297 nm and, with prolonged exposure, it produces chronic effects such as loss of elasticity and carcinoma.

If the eyes are irradiated by UVB photokeratitis may develop after a variable interval depending on the degree of exposure but usually within 6–12 hours. The condition is known as arc eye because it is seen most frequently in those who look at arc welding without protective goggles— rarely the welder. Arc eye is marked by a painful conjunctivitis and blepharospasm which disappears within 24–48 hours. In the most severe cases the patient may be photophobic for a few days after the incident. The eyes do not develop a tolerance to repeated UV exposure so they must always be protected. Intense UV irradiation may induce the formation of cataracts and there is a suggestion that the cataracts found in furnace-men and others exposed to red heat may be caused by UV rather than infra-red radiation. Exposure to solar UV radiation may be responsible for a gradual yellowing of the lens and for the production of senile cataracts.

Exposure standards

Maximum permissible exposures for UVA are expressed in units of Joules per square metre (J/m^2) or in irradiation units of watts per square metre. The limits for the eye and skin for periods of exposure exceeding 10^3 seconds are 10^4 J/m^2 or 10 W/m^2. For UVB, the limits vary according to wavelength. If exposure is to a broad band of UV—as is usually the case—the maximum permitted exposure is calculated from the sum of the relative irradiance from each spectral component, each being weighted by a factor known as the relative spectral effectiveness which is taken as 1.0 for a wavelength of 270 nm. The effective irradiance, E_{eff}, is expressed in W/cm^2. Permissible exposure times per day vary from 8 hours when E_{eff} is 10^{-3} to 10 minutes at 5×10^{-2} and 0.01 seconds when E_{eff} is 3×10^2.

Infra-red radiation

IR radiation has a wavelength in the range 700 nm to 1 mm. Its biological effects lie not only in its capacity to heat the tissues by which it is absorbed (the skin and the eye), but also because it can also excite vibration in large molecules which releases emissions of UV; hence those exposed to red heat receive both UV and IR radiation.

Radiation in the range 400–1400 nm is transmitted through the eye and focussed on the retina. Since it is difficult to look at a bright light for more than a few milliseconds, the eye is protected from the effects of IR. If this aversion reflex is overcome, however, severe retinal burns may be produced and since the radiant energy is focussed on the most sensitive part of the retina, the injury can have a catastrophic effect. IR radiation with a wavelength greater than 1400 nm can burn the corneal epithelium; the iris is susceptible to radiation with a wavelength of 1300 nm and the lens is sensitive to two bands, 1400–1600 and 1800–2000 nm. Long term exposure to IR can produce cataracts because of the increase in temperature in the tissues of the eye which results from absorption. Skin burns may occur at all wavelengths but most people remove themselves from exposure when the skin becomes uncomfortably hot, before any serious damage occurs.

Microwave and radio frequency radiation

This is defined as radiation having a wavelength in the range 1 mm to 30 km (or a frequency in the range 0.3–300 000 MHz). The main use of

MW/RF radiation is in providing a source of heat (as in microwave cookers or heat sealing operations) and in communications. It is the thermal properties of MW/RF radiation which provide the principal risk to health; cataract formation is discussed elsewhere. Local irradiation may cause burns whilst whole body irradiation can induce thermal stress which, if sufficiently severe, may cause death. Such deaths have been produced in animals which have been experimentally exposed to continuous-wave whole body irradiation but no undisputed human case has been reported.

In the countries of eastern Europe it is widely held that low levels of MW/RF radiation can cause a variety of non-thermal effects including changes in behaviour. None of these effects has been recognized in the west where the exposure limit of 10 mW/cm^2 is several orders of magnitude higher than that in the eastern bloc countries.

Lasers

A laser is a device which is used to generate high-intensity beams of electro-magnetic energy; the word laser is an acronym for light amplification by stimulated emission of radiation. The device is used to generate a high energy beam of coherent radiomagnetic energy and has three basic components, the active medium, an energy source and a resonant optical cavity. The active (laser) medium contains a population of atoms of molecules which can be raised to a high energy level from the normal ground energy level; in this so-called inverted state, the atoms or molecules can be stimulated to emit photons of the same energy and all in phase. To raise the electrons to high energy levels in a laser, a pumping system is necessary. The pumping system supplies energy to the laser medium until population inversion occurs. There are many pumping systems available including optical, electron collision and chemical reaction. In optical pumping systems, a strong light source is used such as a xenon flashtube or another laser such as a nitrogen or an argon laser. Electron collision pumping is achieved by passing an electric current through a laser medium which may be a gas (as in the case of the helium–neon laser) or a semiconductor junction (as in the gallium arsenide laser). Alternatively, electrons may be accelerated in an electron gun to impact on the laser material. Chemical pumping is based on the energy released during the making or breaking of chemical bonds; some hydrogen fluoride and deuterium fluoride lasers are pumped in this way.

The optical cavity is formed by placing mirrors at each end of the laser medium so that the beam of radiation is passed through the medium several times in order to amplify the number of protons in the medium. One of the mirrors is only partially reflecting so that part of the beam is permitted to escape from the cavity; the geometry of the mirrors determines the shape of the emitted laser beam.

Lasers are generally known by the type of medium which is employed. Thus, they may be solid-state (in which a glass or crystalline medium is used), gas, semiconductor or liquid (in which an organic dye is used). Lasers may operate continuously, in which case they are termed continuous wave lasers and the beam irradiance is constant with time; alternatively they may operate in pulses, delivering repetitive pulses of energy, the duration of which vary from a few milliseconds to fractions of a microsecond.

Lasers may emit radiation in the ultra-violet, visible light of infra-red spectra and the hazard which is presented by a particular type of laser is dependant upon which is emitted; as expected, however, the target organs are the skin and the eye. Great care must be taken when using lasers that appropriate control is exercised; if the radiation emitted is outside the visible spectrum an aiming beam should be incorporated so that the position of the laser beam can be inferred. Locks must be included in the design of the laser so that the instrument cannot be switched on accidentally and the device should be used only by authorized personnel. All workers involved with lasers should be issued with and wear the appropriate safety goggles and when used for surgery, the patient must be protected. For CO_2 lasers (which emit IR) cotton wool pads soaked in saline can protect the patient's eyes and saline soaked clothing may be required for the rest of him. It should be noted that CO_2 lasers can set dry cotton or paper drapes on fire and this must be taken into account when using them in the operating theatre. For all uses, a local code of practice must be established and a laser safety officer should be appointed.

Maximum permissible exposure limits (MPELs) have been recommended for both direct exposures and for exposure from a diffuse reflection of a laser beam. The MPELs are expressed in terms of the radiance (in watts or Joules/cm^2) falling on the cornea. On the basis of the type and energy of their emissions, it is possible to put lasers into four classes:

Class 1: These are the lowest powered lasers and are not considered hazardous if they are incapable of damaging the eye or burning the skin.

Class 2: Only lasers which emit visible light (within the spectrum 400–700 nm) fall within this class and they are considered to be low-risk because damage to the eye will occur only if the normal aversion response to bright light is overcome. Since there will always be a few people who will force themselves to stare fixedly into an intensely bright light for a minute or two, lasers in this class should bear a label to warn of the dangers of this practice.

Class 3: Lasers in this class are moderate risk because they can cause damage to the retina within the natural aversion response time (about 0.25 seconds). They do not cause serious skin damage and their diffuse reflections are not dangerous under normal use. The safety precautions which must be taken in their use, however, are often considerable.

Class 4: These are the lasers of highest power and most risk. They may cause serious injury to the skin by direct exposure and their diffuse reflections may cause damage to the eye. In addition, class 4 lasers present a serious fire risk.

NOISE

There are many occupations in which the daily exposure to noise may impair hearing or reduce efficiency, or both. The intensity of sound is expressed in terms of the square of the sound pressure. By convention the units are in steps or ratios of tenfold intensity, each unit known as a bel. For practical purposes units of one-tenth of a bel, the decibel (dB) are used.

On instruments used to measure sound the zero point on the scale is taken as being equal to a sound pressure of 0.0002 micro bars, the weakest sound pressure which can be detected by a child under very quiet conditions. With any given sound pressure, however, the response varies with the frequency of the sound, maximum sensitivity occurring between 1000 and 4000 cycles per second or Hertz(Hz). The auditory field lies between 20 and 20,000 Hz but the threshold of differentiation between two sounds varies with frequency, each frequency having specific maximum and minimum audibility thresholds. Between 1000 and 4000 Hz the differential threshold varies very little and this is the zone of maximum sensitivity to sound intensity. The threshold of audibility is at its minimum at 4000 Hz and at this frequency is located the zone of impairment of high pitched tones that occur in the very early stages of hearing loss.

When measuring sound, allowance is made for the variation in response to sound of different frequencies. Sound level meters incorporate electrical circuits, known as weighting networks, which provide for variation in sensitivity to sound of different frequencies, the objective being to simulate the characteristics of the ear. A number of scales are in use, but the A weighting is the one generally used for descriptive purposes and sound levels are reported in dB(A). Some typical sound levels are shown in Table 9.5.

The acoustic reflex

The ear is protected to some extent from noise by the acoustic reflex. In response to loud sounds, the stapedius and tensor tympani muscles contract, with the result that less energy is transmitted to the sound receptors of the inner ear. The protection afforded is limited by muscle fatigue and by the delay in response so that it is impossible to cope with sudden, unexpected sounds.

Auditory fatigue and masking

Auditory fatigue and masking are physiological effects noted on exposure to noise. Auditory fatigue causes a temporary shift in threshold with a consequent decrease in hearing. As the intensity of the sound increases, auditory fatigue becomes more marked and may be associated with tinnitus. It is greatest at 4000 Hz.

Recovery may take several hours, especially if the threshold has risen by more than 50 dB. Pure tones have more effect than broadband noise, and intermittent sounds more than continuous sound. In individuals with a high susceptibility towards a temporary threshold shift there appears to be an association with occupational hearing loss.

Table 9.5. Sound levels of some sources of noise

Source	Level dBA	
Conversation	60	Quiet
Light traffic at 30 m	66	Moderately loud
Dishwasher	76	
Key-punch machine	82	
Milling machine	90	Very loud
Bench lathe	95	
Newspaper press	101	
Textile loom	112	Uncomfortably loud
Pneumatic drill	122	
Aircraft carrier jet deck	140	Painfully loud

Masking refers to the process whereby the threshold of hearing of one sound is raised by the presence of another. The effect becomes more noticeable as the frequencies of the two sounds approach each other. Masking can interfere with the understanding of speech and this can have important repercussions in industry, limiting communication or threatening safety.

Hearing loss

Occupational hearing loss represents the transition from a temporary threshold shift to one which is permanent and it usually has a gradual and often unsuspected onset; it should not be forgotten, however, that severe acoustic trauma such as that experienced in an explosion, may cause immediate deafness by rupturing the ear drum, disrupting the ossicles and damaging the inner ear. The first sign of occupational hearing loss is usually a slight impairment of hearing, detected by audiometry in the 4000 Hz range, spreading at a later stage to the 3000–6000 Hz range (Fig. 9.2). This characteristic pattern allows occupational hearing loss to be differentiated from other forms of

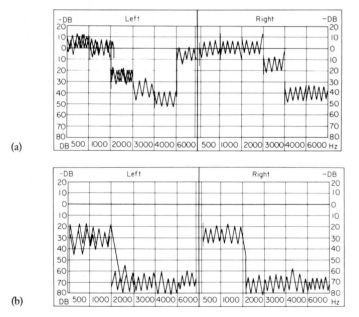

(a)

(b)

Fig. 9.2. Audiograms showing mild (a) and more extensive (b) hearing loss of occupational origin.

deafness. The patient may be completely unaware of any defect in hearing until the speech frequencies are affected. The speech frequencies lie between 500–2000 Hz and may be sub-divided into vowel (500–1000 Hz) and consonant frequencies (1000–2000 Hz).

When hearing loss occurs in these frequencies, speech becomes increasingly difficult to understand, and the patient suffers from some degree of social handicap. It may take years for deafness of this severity to develop but there is no possibility of its reversal since it implies permanent damage to the organ of Corti.

Impulse noise is the most dangerous form; gunfire being notorious for damaging the hearing of those behind the rifles. The intermittent noise of drop-forging is another source which can lead to a rapid deterioration in hearing.

Aetiology of occupational deafness

The ultimate site of the damage induced by noise is the sensory hair cells on the basilar membrane of the cochlea but why the damage is restricted to a relatively small region of the basilar membrane (that which responds most sensitively to 4000 Hz) is not clear. It has been suggested that noise may induce strong mechanical forces along the organ of Corti which physically shake the cells of the membrane and that the 4000 Hz area on the membrane is most susceptible to physical damage. Other authorities have noted that intense noise stimulation induces vasoconstriction in the capillaries in the cochlea which reduces the supply of oxygen and nutrients to the hair cells; under this theory, the cells at 4000 Hz would be inherently more sensitive to this deprivation than cells in other areas.

Nonauditory effects of noise

Noise has been shown to produce effects on the body in addition to causing hearing loss. The heart rate is modified in response to noise, being either increased or decreased depending on the type of noise, and the respiratory rate often increases. Cardiac output is generally decreased and peripheral vaso-constriction may cause blanching of the skin in some people.

All these changes reflect a response on the part of the adrenal gland or the autonomic nervous system to the noise stimulus analogous to those demonstrated by someone who is frightened, and it is unlikely that they are specifically caused by the noise but rather by the individual's reaction to it. None of these changes is permanent and the suggestion that men exposed to noise are more likely than average to develop hypertension has not been confirmed.

Psychological effects

Noise can affect the performance of psycho-motor tasks either adversely or beneficially depending upon its intensity, frequency, duration and intermittence. Sudden, unexpected noise always interferes with the performance of a task, whether mental or physical. Canned music is often introduced into works and other situations with the notion that it engenders a sense of well-being and improves efficiency. Some studies appear to bear out this assumption. Many individuals, however, find that such intrusions are annoying and that they interfere with their performance. The attitude to noise at work seems largely determined by the significance which the individual attaches to it.

Noise and mental illness

There is little reliable evidence that there is any connection between noise and neurotic illness although some categories of neurotic patients show responses to noise which are markedly different from those of normal subjects. For example, hysterical patients fail to habituate noise whilst anxious patients will show a much greater than normal adrenal response.

Deafness is associated with significantly higher rates of mental illness in the community and in hospital populations. In the elderly, deafness is likely to be associated with paranoid states, whereas in young patients, affective disorders are more common. Deafness acquired during late childhood or early adult life causes a profound change in life style and leads to an increased feeling of isolation. The deaf are treated with much less sympathy by their fellows than the blind, and this may help foster the sense of isolation.

Since noise may induce deafness, it can thus be said to have a secondary effect on mental illness.

Hearing conservation

There are many components to a hearing conservation programme, including the reduction of noise at source, limiting exposure with or without ear protectors, and routine monitoring of the workplace and of the work population exposed.

Reducing noise at source can be achieved by enclosing noisy areas with sound insulating partitions, by silencing exhaust systems, and by enclosing noisy machines, or by enclosing the operator of a noisy machine in an insulated box. When choosing new machinery or deciding which of a number of different processes to use, the industrialist should take noise control into account as an important factor in making his decision.

Exposure to noise in an 8 hour day should not exceed a level of 90 dB(A), assuming the noise is relatively steady. Where the sound fluctuates, then the equivalent continuous sound level for an 8 hour shift must not exceed 90 dB(A). In some circumstances it may be difficult to measure and control noncontinuous exposure, as, for example, when a man moves from one area of the factory to another. In these circumstances any exposure exceeding 90 dB(A) should not be allowed.

When ear protectors are worn, noise levels greater than 90 dB(A) are permissible so long as the noise is reduced by the protectors below this level. Under no circumstances whatever must the unprotected ear be exposed to steady levels greater than 135 dB, or in the case of impulse noise, to levels greater than 150 dB.

To comply with these requirements, which are contained in the Code of Practice produced by the Department of Employment, routine noise monitoring has to be undertaken, and noisy areas should be clearly identified with posters, warning of the need to use ear protectors.

Ear protectors are of several forms and they vary considerably in their ability to cut out noise. The simplest forms are ear-plugs, either re-usable rubber or plastic plugs which come in several sizes, or disposable plugs fashioned from 'acoustic wool'. For the re-usable plugs to be effective, they must be of a correct size and make a good seal in the auditory canal. Care must be taken to keep them clean by regular washing. Acoustic wool is extremely fine glass fibre which can be formed to make a plug for insertion into the ear. It is discarded after use. The wool comes in dispensers which automatically supply the correct amount to make a plug. It is cheap and effective but some people develop an eczematous reaction to the glass fibre which may require them to discontinue its use. Cotton wool is an extremely poor protector and should not be used.

The most effective form of protection is the earmuff of which there are two varieties, those with a liquid seal and those with a seal of soft plastic foam. The degree of protection they afford is tested by audiometry and their efficiency varies according to the frequency of the sound (Table 9.6). Their main disadvantage is that they are uncomfortable because they are sweat-traps and men cannot always be persuaded to continue with them, preferring the less effective ear-plugs.

Table 9.6. Typical performance of fluid seal ear muffs*

Frequency	Hz	125	250	500	1000	2000	4000	8000
Mean attenuation	dB	13	20	33	35	38	47	41
standard deviation	dB	6	6	6	6	7	8	8
Assumed protection	dB	7	14	27	29	31	39	33

*The assumed protection is the sound reduction given to the majority of users, and is obtained by subtracting the standard deviation from the mean attenuation.
From Department of Employment Code of Practice for Reducing the Exposure of Employed Persons to Noise, HMSO, 1972.

Routine audiometry is often used to monitor hearing loss in individuals exposed to noise, the results being compared with those of a test performed before the man was exposed. It would be clearly unwise for an individual who already has some hearing deficit to be employed in a job which entails some risk of further deterioration. Many firms now use audiometry programmes on their employees and apparatus is available which enables the man under test to administer it himself.

Ultrasonic and infrasonic noise

Ultrasonic waves are those generated at frequencies above the limit of human hearing. They occur in the range from about 16 KHz up to about 10M Hz. Ultrasound has a number of industrial applications including cleaning and welding plastics, drying fine powders, emulsification and detecting flaws in materials. It is also becoming increasingly used in medicine, mainly in the fields of obstetrics, cardiology, neurology and ophthalmology.

It has been suspected that ultrasonic waves may lead to the local generation of heat in biological materials. Experimental studies have shown that tissue damage can result from ultrasound but follow-up studies of mothers and fetuses have not revealed this to be a hazard in obstetric use.

Hearing loss and vasoconstriction have been reported concomitants of its industrial use, but some effects attributed to ultrasound have been blamed on sound in the high frequency audible range.

Infrasound, such as is generated by diesel engines, generators and turbo-jet and rocket engines has been shown to produce dramatic effects in exposed subjects. Vertigo and nausea are caused by the excitation of the semi-circular canals and the vibrations may produce resonance in the internal organs producing a sensation of discomfort. Vibrations in the chest wall may induce changes in respiration. Subjective symptoms such as headache and fatigue have been recorded.

Careful experimentation using human volunteers has indicated that men wearing ear protectors can tolerate noise in the 1–100 Hz range for short duration even when the sound pressure levels are as high as 150 dB. For the frequency range above 40 Hz, however, such exposure approaches the limits of tolerance.

VIBRATION

Vibrating tools may give rise to injury to the soft tissue of the hands and cause pains in the joints of the arms, most commonly the elbows and wrists. Workers using pneumatic tools and chain saws are commonly found to have small cysts and vacuoles and osteoporotic changes in the bones of the wrist on X-ray examination. These are usually symptomless and do not give rise to any complaint. The other common disorder, however, is vibration induced white finger. This condition occurs in a variety of occupations and all those who use pneumatic tools or rotating tools for grinding and other purposes are potentially at risk. Chain saw operators are a high risk group who have been intensively studied in recent years.

Vibration induced white finger (VWF) takes several years to develop as a rule and is commonly preceded by tingling and numbness in the fingers. Blanching is first noticed in 1 or 2 fingers in the winter but as the condition progresses, all the fingers become involved and episodes of blanching occur in both winter and summer. The condition can be arbitrarily divided into a number of stages for descriptive purposes (Table 9.7).

The mechanism by which the changes found in VWF are induced is not clearly understood. Arteriograms of affected patients show that the proximal segments of the digital arteries may be occluded but the occlusion is related to attacks of finger blanching only to the extent that the degree of occlusion affects the blood flow through the finger. Thus, reducing the blood flow will make the finger more susceptible to the effect of cold, but this, in itself, does not produce the blanching effect.

Histologically, the occluded arteries show marked medial hypertrophy and fibrosis with extreme intimal thickening and elastosis. These changes reduce the size of the lumen but the final obliteration often results from thrombosis and the organization of the thrombus.

There is no doubt that during an attack of white finger the circulation of the finger has ceased but, as already mentioned, arterial occlusion does not cause blanching of the skin, rather it is due to the loss of blood from the sub-papillary venous plexuses. Finger-tip blood flow is diminished in response to cold in users of vibrating tools, whether or not they have VWF, but in contrast to normal subjects, there is no subsequent phase of cold dilatation. Various hypotheses have been put forward to explain this phenomenon, including failure of local biochemical regulations due to damage to the vessel wall or nerve endings in the fingers. The fact that the condition frequently progresses even when the man changes his work, suggests that the damage sustained is permanent. The more popular hypothesis is that the damage sustained by nerve endings is the most significant, but an alternative point of view holds that the formation of callus in the finger pads eliminates the reservoir of blood which is normally present in the small blood vessels and which is necessary to accommodate sudden changes in blood volume.

Table 9.7. Stages of vibration induced white finger

Stage	Condition of Digits	Work and Social Interference
O	No blanching of digits	No complaints
O_T	Intermittent tingling	No interference with activities
O_N	Intermittent numbness	
1	Blanching of one or more fingertips with or without tingling and numbness	No interference with activities
2	Blanching of one or more complete fingers with numbness usually confined to winter	Slight interference with home and social activities. No interference at work
3	Extensive blanching usually all fingers bilateral. Frequent episodes summer as well as winter	Definite interference at work, at home and with social activities. Restriction of hobbies
4	Extensive blanching. All fingers; frequent episodes summer and winter	Occupation changed to avoid further vibration exposure because of severity of signs and symptoms

The question as to whether VWF progresses to produce the clinical features associated with Raynaud's phenomenon is still a matter for some dispute. Most authorities, however, incline to the view that

Raynaud's phenomenon of occupational origin is a definite entity and patients have been described with severe trophic changes in the hand, including gangrene, apparently as the result of their work. Despite this, the Industrial Injuries Advisory Council has declined to recognize this disease as qualifying for industrial compensation.

Prevention

A number of countries, including the USSR, Czechoslovakia and Japan have regulations governing the use of vibrating tools. In Great Britain, the British Standards Institute has produced draft recommendations but as yet there are no regulations. The British Standards Institute recommendations are based on the acceleration produced in m/sec^2 in a wide range of frequencies and on the time and type of exposure. For a 5 hour period of continuous exposure, or an 8 hour period of interrupted exposure the maximum acceleration allowed is shown in Table 9.8.

Table 9.8. Maximum accelerations recommended in each frequency range in vibrating tools*

Frequency	Up to 16	31.5	63	125	250	500	1000	2000
Maximum acceleration m/sec^2	1	2	4	8	16	32	64	128

*BSI Draft Recommendations.

For exposure of shorter duration, greater accelerations may be permitted. Where this is less than 30 minutes continuous exposure, then the values in Table 9.8 may be increased by a factor of 10.

Whole body vibration

Mechanical vibration between 5 and 11 Hz will cause the body to resonate. Exposure to vibration of this frequency occurs in bus, truck and tractor drivers and in helicopter and aeroplane pilots. Whole body vibration is thought to predispose to back pain and changes in the lumbar and thoracic vertebrae have been recorded. In the United States, prostatitis seems to be a particular hazard amongst army drivers who refer to the condition as jeep drivers' disease.

Sick building syndrome

This is an inaccurate and inelegant term which is applied to the symptoms which may be experienced by those who work in new, or newly renovated, buildings. It is characteristic that the building is entirely artificially lit and air conditioned so that it is impossible for the worker to open a window, alter the temperture or change the lighting. The symptoms invariably occur in epidemics and those most commonly complained of include headaches, irritation of the eyes, nose and throat, pains in the joints or muscles, fatigue, and tightness in the chest. The symptoms are generally thought by the patients to be caused by some contaminant in the environment, perhaps coming from the air conditioning system. They may begin after urea-formaldehyde insulating foam has been installed. In many cases the most extensive surveying of the environment reveals no abnormality other than low humidity and the symptoms may remit when the humidity is increased; sometimes altering the lighting also has a beneficial effect. This condition can be clearly distinguished from humidifier fever and the air conditioning is generally blameless if it is not sending round air which is too dry. If urea-formaldehyde foam is installed badly there may be a leakage of formaldehyde from cracks in the walls or around window frames or central heating pipes and the concentration of gas may be sufficient to produce conjunctivitis and irritation of the upper respiratory tract. The concentration of formaldehyde rapidly falls as the foam hardens, however, but symptoms noted after the event may be considered to have been caused by the gas. In a small number of cases, patients appear to have become sensitized to formaldehyde or to dust from the foam and they develop asthma.

In the majority of cases no external agent can be found to account for the symptoms and it is most probable that workers are somatising their dislike for an environment over which they have no control. There is obviously an overlap between this syndrome and mass hysteria and it can be a most difficult condition with which to cope.

CHAPTER 10/INFECTIOUS DISEASES

Dirt in one form or another is an inevitable accompaniment of many forms of work and thus sepsis following accidental cuts at work is common. For this reason employees in many factories are encouraged to have courses of immunization against tetanus.

In some occupations there is a considerable risk from general infections, medical and veterinary practice being outstanding examples. Workers in laboratories in which micro-organisms are handled for diagnostic or experimental purposes are also at risk and in an attempt to contain this risk, a strict code of practice must be adhered to. Pathogens can be classified according to the risk they present and the precautions taken when handling them vary accordingly. Four risk categories have been proposed, as follows:

Group 1: A biological agent that is most unlikely to cause human disease;

Group 2: A biological agent that may cause human disease and which might be a hazard to laboratory workers but which is unlikely to spread in the community at large. Laboratory exposure rarely produces infection and effective prophylaxis or treatment are available;

Group 3: A biological agent that may cause severe human disease and present a serious hazard to laboratory workers. It may also present a risk of spread within the community but effective prophylaxis or treatment are usually available; and

Group 4: A biological agent which has all the properties of Group 3 organisms but for which there is usually no effective prophylaxis or treatment.

The majority of pathogenic bacteria fall into Group 2 whilst all the *Rickettsiacae* are put into Group 3. Most fungi are Group 2 organisms as are most parasites. All viruses are classified as at least Group 2; the hepatitis B virus is a Group 3 pathogen whilst the viruses which cause haemorrhagic fever are in Group 4.

Specific infectious disease of occupational origin are relatively few in number; those which are most serious or which occur most commonly are discussed below.

191

Hepatitis B

There are three known forms of viral hepatitis, A, B, and non-A, non-B; hepatitis B is the only form which presents an occupational risk, particularly to hospital staff and others whose work brings them into contact with blood or blood products. The risk from hepatitis B was highlighted during the rapid introduction of renal dialysis units when there were several cases in the staff of the units, some of them fatal. In due time, a code of practice was evolved which has considerably diminished the risk to staff in renal units.

Contact with the virus is most often brought about by inocculation injuries or when blood comes into contact with mucous membranes, following a splash of blood in the eyes, for example. The incubation period varies between 30–150 days and the symptoms of the disease include malaise, myalgia, headache, nausea, vomiting, anorexia, abdominal pain and pruritus. The patient becomes jaundiced, passing dark urine and pale stools, and the liver may be tender and enlarged. Liver function tests will be wildly abnormal; the diagnosis is confirmed by demonstrating the presence of surface antigen (HBsAg). The normal course of events is that the patient will show a brisk antibody response and recover completely. At the end of the illness, the patient will retain a relatively high antibody (HBAB) titre but will be antigen negative. A proportion of patients will become carriers, however, and some may develop chronic hepatitis.

Prevention: All staff who work in renal units should be screened for the presence of HBsAg and those found to be positive employed elsewhere. Patients who are antigen positive should be dialysed away from the main unit and donor blood should also be screened and not used if it is antigen positive. There is now an effective hepatitis B vaccine which may be offered to staff considered at high risk after appropriate screening; they would not require the vaccine if they were already HBAB positive. The experience to date is that there is an extremely low take-up of the vaccine until an accident occurs involving a patient who is antigen positive.

In all hospitals (and other places where contact with the virus is possible) there must be a procedure to deal with inocculation injuries. No matter how seemingly trivial they should be reported as quickly as possible after the event and an attempt must be made to identify the patient whose blood contaminated the sharp instrument. If this can be done, then the antigen status of the patient is determined; if it is negative, then no more need be done except to give advice on the safe handling or disposal of sharps. If the patient is positive then blood must be taken from the person having had the accident and his antigen and antibody status determined. If the accident took place within 4 weeks, then immunoglobulin may be given; if it is more than 4 weeks since the accident occurred, immunoglobulin is ineffective. Vaccination can be offered providing the interval between the injury and the proposed date of starting the course of vaccination is less than 6 weeks. There is as yet insufficient clinical evidence to be able to determine whether or not vaccination during the later stages of the incubation period will cause a fulminating type of disease which would be worse for the patient than allowing the disease to run its natural course. It is for this reason that all accidents must be promptly reported.

Although medical and nursing staff may be at risk from contracting the disease from their patients, there have been few instances in which it has been shown that antigen positive doctors or nurses have infected their patients. A few outbreaks of hepatitis have been traced to dentists but this risk can be minimized if the dentist wears gloves when he is working, since infection usually results from the leakage of serum from small lacerations on the hand into the patient's mouth. In a very few cases, hepatitis B has been transmitted from surgeons to their patients as a result of blood from the surgeon getting into the wound following a laceration on a scalpel or needle. Scrupulous attention to technique and wearing an additional pair of gloves have been found to eliminate the risk. There is at present a misconception amongst medical and surgical staff that if they were found to be antigen positive this would lead to their sudden and premature retirement. This is not so and shows a curious, not to say complacent frame of mind. An antigen positive surgeon does not pose less of a risk to his patients because he does not know he is antigen positive; indeed, by knowing, he is much more likely to be safer since he will then take greater care when operating.

One other preventive method which can be employed is to screen all high risk patients when they are admitted to hospital; if any are found to be antigen positive then the hospital staff can be forewarned to take extra care when taking blood or giving any form of treatment which necessitates the use of knife or needle.

Anthrax

Anthrax is the result of infection with the *Bacillus anthracis*, a gram-positive, spore-forming organism. The spores are extremely resistant and can survive for long periods in the soil and in animal remains. Cattle are the main reservoir of infection, but these days, imported foodstuffs such as bone and fish meal account for most cases. All those handling infected meat, hides and skin, wool or other animal products are potentially at risk. Workers in bone meal factories are probably the group with the highest exposure and cases have occurred in gardeners handling infected bone meal. Hides and skins, wool and hair imported from the Far and Middle East are notorious for their potential to transmit the infection.

Three varieties of the disease occur, cutaneous, pulmonary and gastro-intestinal, the last two being rare in this country, the g–i form very rare.

Cutaneous anthrax

This form of the disease usually occurs on an exposed part of the body and is caused by spores from infected material gaining entry through cuts or abrasions on the skin. The condition is sometimes referred to as malignant pustule, but this is an inaccurate description since the lesion is rarely malignant and never pustular. In three-quarters of all cases the lesions occur on the face, head and neck.

After an incubation time of 1–4 days a small, irritant red papule develops which rapidly becomes vesicular and necrotic in the centre forming a characteristic black eschar. This lesion may be surrounded by a ring of secondary vesicles from which *B. anthracis* can be cultured. Pain is not common, but itching is. Widespread nonpitting oedema often surrounds the lesion but lymph node involvement is rare. Constitutional symptoms and fever are usually absent unless the skin infection is severe or the infection becomes disseminated, when pyrexia, collapse and death are all possible events. In cases where the lesion is on the face or neck, the intense oedema may threaten life.

The disease can usually be diagnosed on clinical grounds and by the culture of fluid obtained from the vesicles or from under the eschar. Blood cultures should also be made. Serological tests are available if necessary, the best known being Ascoli's test, and fluorescent antibody techniques can also be used for the identification of bacteria in cultures or tissue sections.

Pulmonary anthrax

Pulmonary anthrax was once relatively common amongst workers in the woollen industry and was referred to as 'wool-sorters' disease'. Nowadays, only a very small percentage of cases are of this sort. There is no external lesion and this makes diagnosis difficult. The illness begins abruptly and there are severe toxaemic symptoms. Haemorrhagic mediastinitis with widening of the mediastinal shadow on X-rays and haemorrhagic meningitis may occur. There is widespread pulmonary congestion and oedema with frothy blood-stained sputum. Death is very common in this form of anthrax and the disease may run its complete course in just a few days.

Treatment: Penicillin and tetracycline are both effective, penicillin being the drug of choice. In cutaneous cases recovery is the rule and there is usually no scarring. The pulmonary disease may progress so rapidly that death results even with appropriate treatment.

Prevention of the disease depends upon its eradication in animals. In Great Britain anthrax in cattle is rare and when it does occur the animal is destroyed and the carcase deeply buried or cremated without autopsy, and the rest of the herd is vaccinated. Disease control in other countries is often ineffective and thus it is difficult to prevent the importation of potentially infective material. Regulations exist governing the importation and disinfection of wool and hair but other animal products are exempt. Bone meal is almost impossible to sterilize and men handling it should be protected by wearing gloves and by the downwards ventilation of working surfaces.

Immunization against anthrax is now freely available to those for whom the disease may be an occupational hazard. Three intra-muscular injections of vaccine are given at intervals of 3 weeks, followed by a booster dose 6 months after the third injection. An annual booster is recommended for those who continue at risk. Reactions to the vaccine are rare and when they do occur, are usually mild. Cases of anthrax have not occurred in those who have completed the course of immunization.

Glanders

Glanders, of farcy, is a disease of horses, mules and donkeys, although most warm-blooded animals, except the ox, pig and the white mouse, may become infected. The infecting organism is a gram-negative bacillus variously called *Pfeifferella mallei* or *Bacillus mallei.* Infection in man is now very rare and is the result of contact with an infected animal. Horse-hair is also said to be a potential source of infection. The disease occurs in both an acute and a chronic form.

Acute glanders

There is an incubation period of 2–3 days before the patient experiences symptoms of general malaise, headache, anorexia and joint pains. The site of infection becomes ulcerated and there is a marked lymphangitis. Nodular abscesses form along the lymphatics and these break down to form painful ulcers. There is a marked pyrexia, highest between the sixth and twelfth days after which time a characteristic eruption appears on the face and on the nasal, palatal and pharyngeal mucosae. The lesions begin as erythematous patches which rapidly become papular and then pustular. The pustules ulcerate with the destruction of bone and cartilage to produce a thick, blood-stained purulent discharge. A destructive arthritis may also occur with abscess formation in the muscles.

Diagnosis is difficult, but can be established by a history of contact with horses, by agglutination and/or complement fixation tests, by skin tests and by isolation of the organism.

Chronic glanders

This is rarer even than the acute form of the disease and is characterized by the formation of abscesses, which break down to form destructive, painful ulcers. The lungs may be involved with the production of pneumonia, pleural effusion, lung abscesses and emphysema. The disease runs a long course and an acute phase may supervene at any time.

Treatment: There are reports of sucessful treatment with sulphonamides. Streptomycin, tetracycline and chloramphenicol may all be useful but there is, as yet, little clinical experience of the use of antibiotics in the disease. Treatment should be rigorous since the disease carries a 90 per cent mortality rate.

The disease has ceased to be a public health problem with the identification and destruction of infected animals.

Leptospirosis

Infection with pathogenic leptospires produces a wide variety of clinical signs and symptoms. The disease is transmitted to man from the many animals which act as reservoir hosts, including dogs, cats, cattle and pigs. Seven separate sero-groups of pathogenic organisms are known in Great Britian, *Australis, Autumnalis, Ballum, Canicola, Hebdomadis, Ictero-haemorrhagiae* and *Javanica*. They are not all equally virulent, but the clinical manifestations and the pathological lesions produced by each and their modes of transmission are similar enough to justify considering them all together.

Transmission may occur by direct contact with the blood, tissues or organs of infected animals, the kidneys being the most likely to be infective. More commonly, however, infection occurs from indirect contact with urine. The leptospires have a tendency to persist in the convoluted tubules and to multiply on the epithelium. From this site they are shed in the urine to contaminate the soil, water, or vegetation on which the urine chances to fall.

The occupations which are thought of as being traditionally most at risk, sewer workers, miners and workers in slaughterhouses and fish markets are now seldom affected, and most cases occur in farmers, usually due to *Hebdomadis* infections.

Leptospires can easily pass through intact skin to reach the blood stream. The infection consists of two overlapping phases, leptospiraemia, during which antibodies are produced, and leptospiruria. Symptoms occur mainly in the leptospiraemic phase.

There are no local signs of infection and there is a latent interval of about 7–12 days before the patient develops a fever. At this time the leptospires multiply in the blood and may be carried to and effect any organ.

There are no pathognomonic signs or symptoms and so clinical diagnosis tends to be unreliable. In addition to his fever, the patient may complain of malaise, myalgia, arthralgia, sore throat, conjunctivitis, abdominal pain and tenderness often localized to the right hypochondrium, headache, neck stiffness and photophobia. Conjunctival haemorrhages may aso be noted, together with a macular rash often accompanied by petaechial haemorrhages. Lymphadenopathy and hepatomegaly may be found on clinical examination. Epistaxis, haemoptysis and haematuria when they occur are generally slight, but may be severe enough to require transfusion.

Albuminuria with cells and granular casts are common in the early stages of the disease and are usually transient phenomena but in some cases severe urinary symptoms develop, the blood urea rises and anuria may follow.

There is often mild hepatocellular damage with a moderate increase in transaminase levels, and jaundice may be noted 2–5 days after the onset of fever.

The ESR is invariably raised and there is often an elevation in the white cell count, with a preponderance of polymorphs.

There is usually a steady clinical improvement during the second week of the illness and mild cases recover completely without specific treatment; fatalities are rare unless renal damage is severe.

The diagnosis rests on serological testing: leptospirosis is distinguished in the first place from other causes of fever or jaundice by a complement fixing test using a compound screening antigen. If this is positive, further agglutination tests will identify the serogroup to which the organism belongs.

Penicillin is the treatment of choice, although most other antibiotics are effective, the principal exception being chloramphenicol. Large doses should be used, and treatment begun as early in the course of the disease as possible and continued for 7 days. There are usually no long-term sequelae of the disease.

Erysipeloid of Rosenbach

This disease is caused by a gram-positive organism *Erysipelothrix rhusiopathiae*. It occurs following contact with infected animals or animal products, especially pig, fish and game, but it may also develop in those who handle root vegetables grown in contaminated soil. Those who follow high risk occupations are veterinary surgeons and workers in slaughterhouses and fish or meat markets.

Generally it is a trivial condition, the site most often affected being the finger. Infection occurs through an abrasion on the skin and is signalled by pain and swelling in the affected part. The lesion is red or purple in colour with a sharply-defined margin. It may spread up the finger to the web and descend from there into the next finger. Commonly it spreads onto the dorsum but not the palm of the hand and it seldom extends above the wrist. The pain may be severe but most often is not and there is no throbbing as in pyogenic infection. Lymphgangitis is uncommon. Constitutional symptoms are rare and the lesion rapidly resolves leaving no disability. The lesion is usually sufficiently distinctive to enable a diagnosis to be made without resort to the laboratory.

The disease may in rare cases become generalized and give rise to toxaemic symptoms. In these cases widespread erythema is followed by severe urticaria presenting in the form of rhomboid shaped lesions, 1– 2 cm in size. A bacteraemia form is also known which may be complicated by bacterial endocarditis.

Treatment with penicillin will shorten the duration of the disease but those who contact it know its self-limiting nature and seldom seek treatment. All those who handle material likely to be infected should wear protective gloves, but seldom do.

Ankylostomiasis

This disease is due to the presence of nematode worms in the gut. Man is the natural host for two species of nematode, *Ankylostoma duodenale*, and *Necator americanis*. There is no intermediate host and the ova are excreted in the faeces and hatch in warm moist conditions. The larvae gain entrance to the new host through abraded skin.

Ankylostomiasis is common in the tropics, in southern Europe and in Asia. As an occupational disease it is now an historical curiosity although still one of the prescribed occupational diseases. It was once prevalent in the Cornish tin miners where the hot, moist and insanitary conditions favoured the hatching of the ova (the ovum requires a temperature in excess of 75°C to hatch).

Brucellosis

Brucellosis in man is caused by contact with infected animals. The organism is gram-negative and three species account for most human disease. These species show an affinity for particular animal hosts so that *Br. abortus* is found in cattle, *Br. Melitensis* in sheep and goats and *Br. suis* in pigs.

The disease may occur in men working in slaughterhouses or in those handling meat and meat products. Veterinary surgeons are an outstandingly high risk group. The routes of infection include ingestion, inhalation and direct contact with infected material. Of these, direct contact is the most important and in cases where vets contract the disease, it is usually through handling the placenta or fetal parts during the delivery of a calf. The organism may gain access to the body through abraded skin or through the mucous membranes, including the conjunctiva.

Members of the general public are infected from time to time by drinking raw milk from infected animals, usually when on holiday in the country.

Having entered the body by whatever means, the organisms spread through the lymphatics and lodge in the regional lymph nodes. Entrance to the thoracic duct allows widespread dissemination to take place through the blood stream.

The disease is characterized by the formation of granulomata which occasionally caseate and form abscesses. This happens particularly in infections with *Br. suis*. The organisms are found within monocytes in which situation they are protected to some extent from the action of bacteriocidal antibodies.

Acute brucellosis

The incubation period is variable, from a few days to a few weeks. Onset may be gradual with nonspecific signs and symptoms such as fever, headache, joint pains, insomnia and low back pain, or it may be abrupt with fever, rigors and prostration. The temperature is in the range of 38–40°C but occasional spikes of fever greater than this are found. There are few abnormal clinical findings apart from generalized lymph-adenopathy and a palpable spleen. The peripheral blood count shows a leucopenia with a reduction in the number of polymorphs.

Usually the disease subsides within 2 weeks and the patient makes a complete recovery. Some patients, however, enter a subacute stage and continue to have intermittent bouts of fever, back pain, a feeling of lethargy and depression which may last several months.

Positive blood (or bone marrow) cultures provide the definitive diagnosis but repeated cultures may be necessary as the organism is notoriously difficult to isolate. In most patients, levels of IgM and IgG are raised and both agglutination and complement fixation tests are positive. If a rise in antibody titres can be demonstrated this is good confirmatory evidence for diagnosis. Some patients with positive cultures, however, never develop a positive agglutination or complement fixation test. Conversely, some patients with no evidence of an acute attack of brucellosis nevertheless have persistently raised antibody titres.

Chronic brucellosis

The diagnosis of this condition presents many problems. The main symptoms are like those of the subacute stage, that is, lassitude, headaches, malaise, joint pains and depression of many months duration. Unlike the subacute illness, however, there is by no means always a history of an acute attack. Some patients have serological evidence suggestive of past infection, but serology is unhelpful in making the diagnosis; there is no elevation of IgM or IgG levels as in the acute attack. In many cases the occupation is the only clue which there may be to the diagnosis.

Complications of chronic brucellosis include endocarditis, principally affecting the aortic valve, and spondylitis. The radiological picture in the latter condition may mimic tuberculosis, but can usually be distinguished by the rapid growth of osteophytes from the affected vertebrae which meet to form bridges of lamellar bone. In some patients, chronic, suppurative lesions of the liver and spleen have been described. The lesions usually calcify and the appearance of areas of calcification on an abdominal X-ray may suggest the diagnosis.

Allergy to 'Br. abortus'

Patients with an allergy to *Br. abortus* develop skin rashes or a transient febrile illness with arthralgia following exposure to infected animals or animal products. These patients have a high IgE titre and a strongly positive reaction to the brucellin skin test. They become asymptomatic when removed from contact with infected animals.

Treatment: Tetracycline is the treatment of choice in both acute and chronic brucellosis. It is difficult to achieve a complete cure in chronic brucellosis, however, and long courses of antibiotic therapy are often required. Co-trimaxazole is also effective in both conditions. Streptomycin has no therapeutic value used alone, but may be useful in combination with tetracycline.

The ultimate eradication of the disease depends upon eliminating it in the animal reservoirs and maintaining herds of animals free from the disease.

Q fever

Q fever is a rickettsial infection caused by *R. burneti*. The infection is seen most frequently in farmworkers who usually contract the disease from sheep and cows by the inhalation of infected dust or by the ingestion of raw milk. Veterinary surgeons and abattoir workers constitute other high-risk groups.

The symptoms of the illness are like those of influenza and many cases of Q fever are given this diagnosis. The mistake can be corrected in retrospect when the patient is found to have a raised antibody titre.

Typically the illness begins with the sudden onset of fever accompanied by shivering, sweating and backache. The throat is often inflamed and the conjunctiva are suffused. The patient may complain of photophobia and muscular pain. About half the patients have an unproductive cough. An erythematous rash appears in a few patients.

Patients with a cough often have signs of patchy consolidation and chest X-rays frequently show the presence of single or multiple soft shadows, usually in the lower zones. The consolidation of the chest takes 2–3 weeks to resolve and may be complicated by pleural effusions.

In severe cases headaches and neck stiffness may suggest a diagnosis of meningitis but the cerebrospinal fluid is invariably normal. Lymphadenopathy is sometimes found and pericarditis is a rare complication. Occasionally patients develop signs and symptoms similar to those of sub-acute bacterial endocarditis months, or even years after an acute attack. The organism attacks only valves previously diseased, the aortic valve being most commonly involved.

The diagnosis is suggested by the knowledge that the patient is in a high-risk occupation and confirmation depends upon the presence of a raised antibody titre. Treatment with tetracycline or co-trimoxazole singly or in combination, will produce good results in the acute illness. The results of treatment in cases of endocarditis are poor and the best hope for a cure is with surgical replacement of the damaged valve.

Prophylaxis is difficult because although vaccines are available, animals carrying the organism do not manifest any symptoms so that there is little or no incentive for farmers to maintain Coxiella-free herds.

Orf

Orf is a viral infection of sheep and goats which is occasionally transmitted to those who look after the animals or who handle the meat or its products.

The disease in man, commonly known as contagious pustular dermatitis, takes the form of a mild exanthematous lesion, usually single, occurring at the site of infection. Clinical signs appear 4–12 days after infection, with the development of a red macule or papule. This enlarges until it becomes about 1–4 cm in diameter. It then becomes umbilical and vesicular, containing firstly clear fluid and then pus. There may be some local tenderness and lymphadenitis and the lesion is sometimes painful or itchy. Healing is complete within 4–6 weeks with little or no scarring.

Treatment is symptomatic and the main objective is to secure healing without secondary bacterial infection. The incidence of orf has declined since the introduction of an effective cheap vaccine.

Milkers' nodes

This is a disease of dairy cattle handlers, the infective agent being a virus closely related to the orf virus. It is transmitted from the mouths of calves or from the handling of teats of lactating cows.

The lesion is clinically indistinguishable from orf except that it is not painful, nor does it itch.

Ovine encephalomyelitis

This is a viral disease of sheep which produces a form of cerebral ataxia in affected animals. It is commoner in Scotland and the north of England then elsewhere in Britain. In Scotland it is commonly known as the louping-ill because of the characteristic leaping movements which the diseased animals make. It has been found to occur in shepherds, in farmers, in those engaged in sheep-dipping and in men working in slaughterhouses. The tick, *Ixodus vicinus*, which spreads the animal disease is also responsible for cases in humans with the exception of some laboratory workers who have become infected from cultured material.

The disease has two phases, the first of which lasts about a week, during which time the patient has an influenza-like illness with fever, headache and malaise. Leucopenia is common. This is the viraemic phase and the clinical improvement which follows it lasts for up to a week when the neurotropic phase has its onset. The patient then has fever and meningism with headache, photophobia and neck stiffness. He may vomit, and in severe cases pass into a coma. Physical examination may show signs of ataxia, nystagmus and strabismus due to paralysis of the external rectus muscle. The intracranial pressure may be raised with the cerebrospinal fluid showing a lymphocytosis and a varied protein level.

The disease is usually self-limiting and complete recovery within 3–4 weeks is to be expected.

The diagnosis is usually made in the knowledge of the patient's likely exposure to sheep ticks and these may even be found upon him at the time of examination. Protection from the disease depends upon ridding sheep of the ticks. There is no specific treatment although work is in progress to produce a vaccine with which those at risk could be immunized.

Ornithosis

Ornithosis is a specific infection of birds caused by *Chlamydia psittaci*. Although the disease may occur in all birds, man usually contracts it from those in the order Psittaciformes, and so the disease is frequently called psittacosis regardless of the species of the culprit bird.

The disease is usually transmitted to men through the inhalation of dried, infected droppings, more rarely through contact with the feathers or tissues of infected birds and least often through the bite of an infected bird. It is most usually caught from parrots, parakeets or budgerigars and those at risk include veterinary surgeons, pet shop keepers, pet owners; outbreaks may also occur in poultry workers.

There is a variable incubation period of 7–15 days, and occasionally much longer. The illness is ushered in by slow rise of temperature over the first week. There is a severe headache and malaise with anorexia, myalgia and asthralgia. There is usually a pronounced cough, but it may not appear until the end of the first week. The cough is associated with small amounts of sputum, occasionally streaked with blood. In severe cases, the patient may become delirious and stuporous with signs of extensive pulmonary involvement. Cyanosis will be evident in these cases. Pleuritic signs are rare as are neurological signs. Nausea and vomiting, on the other hand, are common. A macular rash similar to that seen in typhoid has been described, but the spots are smaller. In severe cases jaundice and azotaemia have been reported.

Physical examination reveals relatively few signs. The respiratory rate is rapid and fine crepitations may be heard in the lungs. Changes due to consolidation are only rarely heard. The liver is often slightly enlarged and so also is the spleen. The pulse rate remains low.

Radiographs of the chest may show the presence of areas of patchy infiltration radiating from the hilum, more prominent in the lower zones.

In mild cases the illness lasts only for about a week. In more severe cases it may be up to 3 weeks before recovery is complete and relapses are common.

The diagnosis is usually made on the basis of a rising antibody titre or by the isolation of the organism in specialized laboratories.

Tetracycline is the treatment of choice and early diagnosis and prompt initiation of treatment may be life-saving. Chloramphenicol and penicillin are less effective.

Those who own or sell birds should be warned that sick birds may transmit this disease. If they suspect that either they or their birds have the disease, they should promptly seek advice.

CHAPTER 11/ACCIDENTS AND TRAUMA

ACCIDENTS

Accidents at work are an important cause of personal and national loss, both in terms of loss of lives and loss of working time. In Great Britain there are between 400,000 and 500,000 accidents at work each year. Whilst only a small percentage of these are fatal, this nevertheless represents an annual loss of life which is usual in excess of 1000 (Table 11.1).

Something of the order of twenty million working days a year are lost as the result of accidents at work but, as one might expect, the accident rate shows considerable fluctuations as between different industries. This is illustrated in Table 11.2 where the number of days lost each year per thousand employees at risk is shown. It can be seen from this table that the non-manufacturing industries have by far the highest accident rate and this again is what would be anticipated when one considers that it includes such occupations as coal-mining and fishing, both of which are of such a nature as to render them particularly hazardous. Each of the subgroups in the non-manufacturing category has a high accident rate as shown in Table 11.3.

The overall economic cost of industrial accidents is difficult to compute with any accuracy since it is the sum of at least four separate costs, none of which is capable of precise quantification. The four divisions of the main cost are, those met by the employee, those met by the employer, those met by the community at large, and those met by the state. As a rough estimate, accidents probably cost the victims or their families a total of not less than one hundred million pounds per year, whilst other costs, including lost production, the award of damages, and the provision of hospital and ambulance services, probably accounts for a sum in excess of two hundred million pounds.

The causation of accidents

A number of theories have been elaborated to account for accidents at work, the most influential of which has been that of accident-proneness. This theory states that some people are more liable to have accidents

Table 11.1. Accidents at work in Great Britain, 1961–1970*

	1961	1962	1963	1964	1965	1966	1967	1968	1969	1970
Factories	161 655 (368)	157 600 (351)	168 106 (332)	217 950 (344)	239 158 (358)	241 051 (372)	247 058 (342)	254 454 (359)	266 857 (357)	255 907 (325)
Docks and warehouses	7506 (37)	7220 (36)	7815 (36)	10 207 (40)	10 178 (39)	9952 (41)	10 483 (25)	11 407 (28)	10 963 (27)	8865 (28)
Construction	23 356 (264)	25 338 (281)	28 348 (242)	40 491 (271)	44 381 (230)	45 607 (288)	46 475 (197)	46 569 (238)	44 570 (265)	39 823 (203)
Mines and quarries	191 208 (284)	201 389 (288)	206 234 (295)	201 364 (244)	209 935 (256)	188 909 (191)	169 763 (181)	144 046 (158)	121 402 (126)	93 983 (124)
Agriculture	12 846 (80)	13 553 (71)	14 548 (65)	13 276 (64)	11 839 (49)	10 680 (73)	10 069 (58)	8722 (63)	8783 (70)	7366 (41)
Offices, shops and railway premises	18 000 (28)	18 000 (28)	18 000 (28)	18 000 (28)	17 225 (34)	18 533 (29)	19 903 (16)	19 075 (39)	19 018 (20)	16 871 (32)
Railways	14 233 (167)	12 139 (118)	11 846 (116)	11 064 (96)	9838 (103)	8236 (72)	8003 (78)	6912 (62)	7335 (69)	7625 (68)
Road transport	16 200 (57)	16 400 (55)	16 600 (65)	18 700 (70)	22 700 (86)	22 900 (78)	25 300 (82)	26 700 (90)	26 300 (81)	33 800 (80)
Civil Aviation	30 (24)	27 (17)	25 (12)	17 (12)	22 (13)	35 (27)	28 (19)	14 (8)	6 (3)	15 (13)
Seamen	8817 (154)	8783 (131)	8805 (70)	9090 (90)	8672 (91)	8769 (118)	8361 (94)	8177 (98)	8421 (52)	8491 (71)
Total	453 851 (1463)	460 449 (1376)	480 327 (1261)	540 159 (1259)	573 948 (1259)	554 672 (1289)	545 443 (1092)	526 076 (1143)	513 655 (1070)	472 746 (985)

*Fatal cases are shown in brackets. From Report of the Roben's Committee, HMSC, 1972.

Table 11.2. Accident rates in different industries

Industry	Days lost each year through accidents/10^3 men at risk*
Non-manufacturing	6000
Construction	1800
Transport	1700
Manufacturing	1200
Distributive	800
Service	700
Professions	200

*Means for 5 years, 1968–72.
From Digest of Statistics Analysing Certificates of Incapacity, HMSO.

than others because of some innate physical or psychological characteristics. Another theory which enjoyed a considerable vogue was that all the members of a population at risk had an equal risk, that is to say, the occurrence of accidents was due to pure chance. Yet another accepted that the first accident was due to chance, but that having sustained one accident, the probability of having a second increased or decreased. These are all difficult theories to test by epidemiological means, however, because the basic hypothesis requires that all those in the sample population shall be exposed to the same risk. Research has tended to concentrate, therefore, on assessing the relative risks associated with such factors as age, experience, medical condition and so on.

Age is one of the most frequently investigated factors in accident research and there seems little doubt that there is an increased incidence in the 'teens and early twenties. In the third and fourth decades

Table 11.3. Accident rates in different non-manufacturing industries

Industry	Days lost each year through accidents/10^3 men at risk*
Coal mining	10 700
Agriculture	1100
Fishing	3500

*Means for 5 years, 1968–72.
From Digest of Statistics Analysing Certificates of Incapacity, HMSO.

the number of accidents declines, thereafter rising again slightly until retirement is reached. The high accident rate in the young seems to be due to their lack of experience in the job, although after a year or two, length of service is not related to the accident rate, whereas age is, indicating that some other factors are also at work.

The state of health might well be expected to be at the root of some accidents and in some cases this does seem to be true. Accidents due to the onset of hypoglycaemia in diabetes or to myocardial infarcation in men with coronary artery disease are obvious examples of acute medical states which might cause an accident, but ill health is a much less common precipitant of accidents than is generally supposed. Similarly, although defects in vision or in hearing do sometimes cause accidents, this happens only rarely and the defect is job-specific, that is to say, only jobs where good vision is essential will show a relationship between the accident rate and poor sight; the same is true so far as hearing is concerned. Some personality traits, including extraversion, neuroticism, aggression and anxiety have been suggested as being related in some way to an excess accident rate, but the evidence is a long way from being conclusive or of being of help in accident prevention schemes. Intelligence does not correlate with accident rates.

Some characteristics of the work pattern have been shown to be determinants in accident causation. Accidents occur at a peak when the work rate is fastest and when the rate of productivity is greatest. There are more accidents when the length of a shift is increased, but generally there are fewer accidents on the night shift and at the end of the working week. Factories in which there is a good working relationship between the employees seem to enjoy a lower accident rate than those bedevilled by internal strife, probably because communications are better where there is a good *esprit de corps*.

The effect of environmental factors such as extremes of temperature, poor lighting and noise have all been studied but with inconclusive results and the possible interactions between these variables has not been studied at all.

Accident prevention

The high social and economic cost of accidents requires that all those involved with occupational health work strenuously towards their prevention. It must be realized that the burden for implementing a safety prevention programme has to be shared equally and is not the prerogative of one particular section of the working population.

There are broadly four means by which accidents can be prevented although not all are of equal importance. The most important measure is to inculcate an attitude of mind in those at risk which makes them aware of the necessary to comply with safety measures, including the wearing of safety clothing.

This attitude will only be fostered if the management recognize that the safety of their work force is their responsibility and thus accept the need to support vigorous safety campaigns. Each factory should have a team of safety engineers whose task it is to see to it that due attention is given to all aspects of safety and that safety regulations are complied with. In order that there should be no misunderstanding on the part of men or management, safety rules and safety instructions ought to be set down for each job where some hazard exists. These must be as comprehensive as possible and amended as required in the light of new knowledge. It will fall to the safety engineers to ensure that these rules are implemented and to do so often requires considerable tact and diplomacy if they are not to be seen as acting in some way as an unofficial 'police force', constantly on the watch for malpractice.

Safety regulations and good habits of work are encouraged by propaganda of one kind or another, one of the most popular being the safety poster. To be effective, posters should be placed in areas where their message has some relevance to the work in progress and they should be changed at frequent intervals so that their message does not become so familiar that it is ignored. They should instruct, and emphasize the positive benefits of working safely. Some firms operate incentive schemes whereby areas of the factory compete with each other in a 'safety league' but the utility of such schemes remains to be assessed.

One of the greatest challenges in a safety programme is to ensure the use of safety clothing since it is well known that its mere provision is no guarantee of its use. As mentioned in other parts of this book, safety clothing is often cumbersome and uncomfortable to wear and this is an area which would benefit from a well directed research effort. Some simple considerations, however, often tend to be overlooked. For example, the appearance of the clothing should not be such that the wearer feels embarrassed or ill at ease in it. This is particularly so when considering safety clothing for women at work. For example, the provision of safety glasses with fashionable frames instead of the standard, rather unattractive ones, may be critical in encouraging their use.

Safety clothing must also be designed so that it does not hinder normal activities. The provision of safety boots which are too heavy to allow comfortable walking is not calculated to gain many users. Because those who design and provide safety equipment are not often called upon to use it under working conditions, elementary considerations such as these may be overlooked, although this happens less often when the men are consulted during the design stage.

Two other points about safety clothing remain to be noted; firstly, no one should consider himself exempt from wearing safety equipment in a designated area. If management does not set a good example in this respect then it follows that safety rules will be given less than enthusiastic support. Secondly, men at work must not be out of pocket if they comply with safety regulations. This means that protective clothing should be provided free, or, as in the case of safety shoes, for example, at subsidized rates.

TRAUMA

To the eye

Injuries to the eye are unfortunately commonplace in industry. The most frequent injuries are those caused by foreign bodies, usually splinters or metal. Every time metal strikes metal there is a hazard from flying splinters; this seems so obvious that it is surprising that men disregard the hazard, risking serious injury, or blindness by not wearing goggles, or by using them to protect their foreheads. Grinding and polishing and all forms of metal working entail some risk from eye injuries. Burns caused by splashes of acid or alkali or by molten glass or metal are common events.

Prompt treatment at hospital is required to salvage a burnt eye. Superficial foreign bodies can often be removed in the works surgery (where there is one). Where the foreign body has penetrated the globe its position will have to be located radiographically (always assuming it is radio-opaque) and then removed surgically.

Physical trauma to the eye

The damage sustained by the eye depends upon the direction in which the force of a blow is transmitted. If directed along the axis of the eye, then the lens may be dislocated, partially or completely, with a resultant distortion of vision. If the lens is completely dislocated backwards, it falls into the vitreous leaving the iris unsupported and tremulous (a condition referred to as an irridodonesis). Frontal dislocation results in the lens falling into the anterior chamber and if this happens it may produce secondary glaucoma by interfering with aqueous drainage. Retinal tears may also result from a blow along the axis of the eye. This is especially serious if the macula is damaged since it is likely to leave the patient with sight which is greatly impaired. Less violent blows may result in retinal haemorrhages which are serious only if they overlay the macula. Sometimes the force of the blow may be so great that the optic nerve is 'popped out' of the globe and there is no prospect of repairing this catastrophe. If the force is directed through the iris there may be a little bleeding into the anterior chamber. The blood gravitates to the lower segment forming a hyphaema which usually disperses in a few days. If the accumulated blood blocks the drainage of the anterior chamber, secondary glaucoma will ensue and surgical drainage will be required. The iris root is sometimes completely torn by the force of a blow. This is referred to as iridodialysis and the pupil becomes D-shaped. Such tears seldom heal but, on the other hand, they rarely interfere with vision.

In addition to the damage described above, any blow to the eye may cause a black eye or corneal abrasions, neither of which is serious as a rule. In addition, any perforating injury is liable to become infected and steps must be taken to prevent this from happening.

Patients with damage to the eye should be referred to an ophthalmic unit. Dislocated lenses can be removed and adequate vision restored with spectacles, much as the sight can be given back to a patient with cataracts. The prognosis for patients with retinal tears varies according to the site of the tear. Peripheral tears do not impair normal vision greatly, although there may be some loss of night vision; tears involving the macula can almost invariably be expected to leave some deficit.

Arc-eye

This condition occurs in men engaged in electric arc-welding or gas-welding using oxy-acetylene torches. It comes about from the intense ultra-violet irradiation which is experienced when gazing at the welding site with the naked eye. It may occur, although less commonly, from looking at molten steel or at an unscreened arc-lamp.

There is no immediate sensation apart from a momentary glare. After a few hours, however, coloured lights may be noted around objects in vision due to oedema of the cornea epitheleum. This is followed by symptoms of pain and conjunctival irritation; the patient feels as though he has dust in his eyes and produces copious tears; he is photophobic. The eyes may become suffused and there may be marked blepharospasm.

The condition is self-limiting and simple treatment will relieve the pain. It need never occur if all those at risk wear goggles or visors which conform to the British Standards specifications.

Bursitis

Bursitis occurs whenever there is repeated mechanical trauma over a bursa. The condition arises in a variety of situations and is known by many colloquial names, for example, weavers' bottom, clergymen's or housemaid's knee and hodman's shoulder, affecting respectively the ischial, prepatellar and subacromial bursea. Bursea may be produced in connective tissues which are subject to frequent but unusual movements and these were also well recognized in the past as being associated with specific occupations. Thus came about Covent Garden lump, Billingsgate lump, humpers' lump and deal-runners' shoulder. These occurred over the vertex in the porters in Covent Garden, over the seventh cervical vertebra in fish porters and timber porters and over the upper part of the clavicle and shoulder, also in timber porters. This increasing use of mechanization has relegated most of these conditions to the status of curiosities; fork-lift drivers' bottom remains to be described.

Patients seldom seek medical treatment for this condition unless there is a sudden increase in its fluid content as the result of a blow when the sac may become filled with blood or interstitial fluid. In either event, the sudden increase in fluid content is painful. The bursa may become secondarily infected and require surgical drainage. If the patient complains that the bursa is unsightly he should be warned that unless he changes his occupation it is likely to persist and that it is, in fact, fulfilling a protective function. As a sop to vanity, the bursal sac can be removed but will recur if the patient continues at his old job.

The beat disorders

There are three so-called beat disorders recognized for the purposes of compensation under the Industrial Injuries Act, beat knee, beat elbow and beat hand.

The first two are in effect the results of acute infection in the bursae around the knee joint and in the olecranon bursa, or acute cellulitis in the tissues around these two joints. In some cases bursitis and cellulitis co-exist. In the case of beat knee the condition is found predominantly in those whose job involves a lot of kneeling with repeated minor trauma. It occurs, as one could expect, most frequently in miners. If the skin is wet, then the disease occurs more frequently. Men returning to work from a period of absence, or men unaccustomed to the job, are more likely to contract it than others. In beat elbow the cause can more often be tracked down to a single injury sustained at work.

Beat hand differs from the other two conditions in that it consists only of cellulitis. It is the result of repeated minor trauma to the hand—so that miners again present frequently with it—but it occurs also in other men who work with a pick or shovel. Those with 'soft' hands are most at risk and wet working conditions also favour its appearance.

The signs are those classically associated with infection, that is to say, pain, swelling, redness and heat. In the hand, the palm of the hand and the palmar surfaces of the thumb and fore-finger are most often affected and if uncontrolled the infection may spread to involve the tendon sheaths. The swelling may spread to involve adjacent tissues and if the infection is severe, may affect underlying joints.

Treatment must be prompt and thorough and have as its aim the restoration of completely normal function. This may call for surgical intervention. In uncomplicated cases, a cure should be expected within a month.

Tenosynovitis

This condition is a non-infective inflammation of the tendon sheaths in the forearm or in the musculo-tendinous junction. When confined to the latter site, the condition is sometimes referred to as peritendonitis crepitans. The usual cause is an unaccustomed and arduous use of the muscles of the forearm brought about either by a change of occupation or a return to a familiar job after a period of absence. Rarely is the condition bilateral.

The presenting signs and symptoms include pain, swelling and tenderness, usually with some loss of function. There are no signs of infection. Crepitus may be felt over affected tendons and is pathogonomic. The avid searcher of clinical signs will be able to hear the crackling in the tendon sheaths with the aid of a stethoscope but it is not often necessary to go to such lengths to make the diagnosis.

Rest and splinting of the wrist will cure the condition in the majority of cases. Where simple measures fail, injections of hydrocortisone may succeed.

Writer's cramp

This condition is characterized by painful spasms of the hand or forearm brought about by repetitive muscular activity. The patient loses the ability to coordinate the movements necessary for the performance of his task, although very often other activities requiring fine motor co-ordination, such as tying shoelaces, can be undertaken with ease.

There are no physical concomitants of the disease and there are no pathological abnormalities, and the condition is usually referred to as being psychiatric in origin. This conclusion is supported by the fact that the condition invariably occurs in those patients, often of obsessional nature, whose job depends on their ability to write. The prognosis is not favourable and the patient is seldom referred for psychiatric help although this would seem to be the logical step in view of the presumptive cause. Usually the patient is advised to seek an occupation which does not call for the tasks which precipitate the attack. Before arriving at the diagnosis it is prudent to take advice from a neurologist lest some serious neurological disorder be overlooked.

CHAPTER 12/CONTROL OF
OCCUPATIONAL HAZARDS

Since occupational diseases have specific causes which can be identified, measures can be taken to control them. Once a hazard has been
identified, a number of preventive measures can be taken, including
substitution, enclosure, removal at source, segregation and, what may
broadly be called good housekeeping.

SUBSTITUTION

If one is considering a hazard from a chemical then the most certain way
to eliminate the risk associated with its use is to substitute a non-toxic
material for the poisonous one. There are a number of instances where
this has been done successfully. For example, freon is used instead of
methyl bromide as a refrigerant, phosphorus sesquiphosphide has been
substituted for white phosphorus in match making, and other substances are used as insulatory materials in place of asbestos. In some
instances, however, the toxic material offers so many technical and
economic advantages to the industry using it that legislation is necessary
to implement a substitution. In yet other cases, it is impossible to
eliminate the toxic material because there is no satisfactory alternative.

When considering physical hazards such as noise and radiation,
substitution is, of course, not possible, but machines can be designed to
keep noise to a minimum and to prevent the escape of radiation into
those areas in which men are working.

ENCLOSURE

Processes which are particularly dangerous can be totally enclosed and
then performed mechanically or by an operator using special apparatus
as in the way that radioisotopes are handled.

REMOVAL AT SOURCE

The aim of this method is to prevent toxic dusts or vapours from
entering the breathing zone of the operator by some form of local
exhaust ventilation. The hazard from dust can also be lessened by using

wet methods for drilling and grinding. In order to work effectively, exhaust ventilation systems require to be well maintained and they must be well designed. To offer adequate protection, ventilation systems must remove the airborne particles of respirable size ($< 5\mu$ diameter) and these are often the most difficult to remove.

Segregation

Where it is impractical to completely enclose a process, then exposure may be limited to a small segregated group of workers. The hazard is not eliminated, but by this means, methods of supervision and control are considerably simplified.

Good housekeeping

High standards of cleanliness in the work place ensure that exposure to harmful materials will be kept to a minimum and also encourage workmen to take due care when engaged in potentially hazardous jobs. Adequate ventilation in the work place reduces the risk from toxic materials by assisting removal and by reducing local concentrations through a dilution effect.

Personal hygiene is an important protective measure and workers should be made fully aware of the hazards to which their occupation is exposing them and at the same time they should also be made aware of appropriate safety measures which they can take to reduce the risks. These measures will often include the wearing of protective clothing and it is too often the case that men will not make the fullest use of the protective clothing which is provided for them. Very often workmen complain that protective clothing is uncomfortable to wear and to some extent this criticism is justified. In order to protect against solvents and oil from splashing on the skin, for example, the aprons and other garments must obviously be impervious, but such materials are also impervious to water and so the workmen become hot and sweaty. Goggles and ear-protectors may also be uncomfortable in hot working conditions if the wearer sweats under them. There is every good reason to continue working towards finding protective clothing which is both safe and comfortable, but until this ideal has been achieved, workmen should be strongly urged by management and preferably by their unions that some degree of discomfort is better than a lost eye, deafness or some disability which could have been prevented.

MONITORING

Even when attention is given to all these points an element of risk still remains in many occupations which requires to be controlled by some form of monitoring, either physical or biological.

Physical monitoring

The risk from toxic materials in industry arises principally from the inhalation of airborne particles or vapours. The philosophy underlying physical monitoring is that if the airborne concentration of the substance (or substances) which constitutes the potential risk is kept below some pre-determined level, then no harm will come to the exposed workers. This pre-determined level is known as the threshold limit value (TLV) and in this country a list of TLVs relating to a wide range of toxic materials is published by the Health and Safety Executive (see Appendix). These figures are taken from similar lists compiled by the American Conference of Governmental Industrial Hygienists.

The TLV of a substance represents a time-weighted average concentration which it is reckoned may safely be inhaled over the normal 8 hour working day. Occasional excursions above the TLV are permitted providing that they are compensated for by periods when the concentration is less than the TLV. The TLV automatically governs the magnitude of the excursion permitted (see Table 12.1). Thus, the higher the TLV, the lower the excursion factor.

Table 12.1. Excursion factors permitted above TLV

TLV range mg m^{-3}	Excursion factor
0–1	3
> 1–10	2
>10–100	1.5
> 100–1000	1.25

Where a mixture of substances is present in the atmosphere then as a general rule they are considered as additive and the sum of the ratio of observed concentrations to permitted concentrations should not be allowed to exceed unity. That is to say, if

$$\frac{C_1}{T_1} + \frac{C_2}{T_2} + \frac{C_3}{T_3} \cdots \frac{C_n}{T_n} \leqslant 1$$

when C_1 = observed concentrations and T_1 = permitted concentrations, then the TLV for the mixture is said not to have been exceeded.

Short term exposure limits (STEL) have been proposed for some materials. These are 10 minute time-weighted average concentrations to which workers may be exposed with a minimal risk of suffering acute effects. STELs are higher than TLVs, but the TLV still applies, so that any period of exposure at the STEL must be compensated by periods of exposure to lower concentrations. Some of the STELs were formerly expressed as ceiling values.

For a small number of substances (acrylonitrile, asbestos, carbon disulphide, ethylene oxide, isocyanates, lead, styrene, trichlorethylene, vinyl chloride and coal dust in mines) there are now so-called control limits. These are exposure limits which are contained in Regulations, in Codes of Practice or in Directives of the European Community or which have been adopted by the Health and Safety Executive. They are limits which are considered to be reasonably practicable on scientific, medical and engineering grounds and they must not be exceeded at any time. There is not the slightest doubt that many more control limits will be introduced in the coming years, especially when the bureaucratic machine of the EEC begins seriously to take action on exposures in the workplace; we may then expect a veritable torrent of directives.

It should be remembered that once an individual has become sensitized to an allergen, there is almost no concentration to which he may be safely exposed and only complete removal from exposure or the most stringent personal protection will be adequate for his safety.

Establishment of TLVs

There are two different approaches to the establishment of TLVs. The first starts from high levels which are known to produce ill-effects and works downwards using increasingly sensitive indices of clinical, biochemical or pharmacological disturbance, using the results as a predictive guide to the development of frank clinical illness. The TLV established by this means will allow some degree of metabolic interference so long as clinical poisoning does not (in general) follow. This approach is the one most often favoured by toxicologists in this country and in the USA.

The second method is to start from a level which is known to produce no change whatever, metabolic or otherwise, and then work upwards using highly sensitive methods to detect the first change from normal. The TLV is then established just below the level which is found to induce a deviation from the normal state of the organism. This approach has found wide acceptance in Russia and the other eastern European countries. The Russian levels are maximum allowable concentrations (MAC) and it is not permitted to exceed them.

Table 12.2. Concentrations of toxic materials in the atmosphere recommended for international use

Substance	Safe concentration* (mg/m³)
Ammonia	20–35
Arsine	0.2–0.3
Beryllium and compounds (as Be)	0.001–0.002
Chlorinated derivatives of diphenyl	1
Chlorinated derivatives of diphenyloxide	0.5
Dinitrobenze	1
Dinitrotoluene	1–1.5
Ethanol	1000–2000
Ferrovanadium	1
Hydrogen chloride (hydrochloric acid)	5–7
Hydrogen sulphide	10–15
Iodine	1
Methyl acrylate	20–35
Molybdenum, soluble compounds, dust (as Mo)	4–5
Nitrobenzene	3–5
Ozone	0.1–0.2
Parathion	0.05–0.1
Phosgene	0.4–0.5
Sulphur dioxide	10–13
Sulphuric acid and sulphuric anhydride	1
Trinitrotoluene	1–1.5
Vanadium (as V_2O_5)	
dust	0.5
fume	0.1
Zinc oxides (fumes)	5
Zirconium and compounds (as Zr)	5

*These are exposures which will not, so far as is known, produce any change in the health or fitness of the exposed person during his lifetime. The figures given are used by some authorities as maximum values, and by others as time-weighted average values.

It is not surprising that methods which are based on different concepts produce permissible levels which may vary by anything up to a factor of 10. So diverse are the levels in different countries that a joint ILO/WHO Committee was able to find values for only 24 substances which varied by a factor of 2 or less and which they felt could be recommended for international use (Table 12.2).

Biological monitoring

A number of criticisms can be levelled against the use of atmospheric TLVs as the sole or even principal means of controlling the hazard from toxic materials. For example, the size of the dust particles in the atmosphere is an important factor in determining the risk they represent since particles greater than $5-7\,\mu$ in diameter are unlikely to penetrate to the alveoli and will not be absorbed. As a rule, however, the TLV does not take account of particle size. Nor does it make any allowance for undue susceptibility on the part of exposed individuals even though this is well known to be a factor in, for example, exposure to lead, benzene, hydrogen sulphide and DNOC.

It is also possible to be misled by the results of general air sampling. For example, although the overall concentration of pollutants may be less than the TLV, there may be local concentrations in excess of the TLV. Men working in these local conditions may, thus, be subjected to an unsuspected hazard. To some extent, this can be guarded against by providing individuals with personal samplers which can be worn during the shift and with which it is possible to make an estimate of individual exposure. Personal samplers may be battery operated; those used for dust sampling invariably so, but for measuring gases or vapours a variety of passive samplers is now available. Passive samplers have a number of advantages over pump driven samplers. In addition to having no electrical parts, they are small and light so that they do not interfere with normal work practices and some types can be put directly into an automatic gas chromatogram for analysis after which they are ready for re-use. Before they can be used in the field, however, a great deal of preliminary work has to be carried out in the laboratory to determine the diffusion characteristics for each gas or vapour which it is proposed to monitor. As yet, passive samplers have relatively few applications but there is no doubt that they will increasingly be used in the future.

Measurements of atmospheric concentrations are a guide to a potential hazard and may serve to draw attention to the need for improved control, but, in order to assess the effects on those exposed, some form

Table 12.3. Suggested maximum permissible values for use in biological monitoring

Chemical	Biological monitor	Normal value	Suggested maximum
Acetone	Blood concentration	< 0.2 mg/dl	2 mg/dl
	Urinary concentration per gram creatinine*	< 2 mg/g	20 mgm/g
Aniline	Methaemoglobin	< 2%	5%
Arsenic	Total concentration in urine	< 10 μg/g	200 μg/g
Benzene	Urinary phenol	< 20 mg/g	45 mg/g
Cadmium	Blood concentration	< 0.5 μg/dl	
	Urinary concentration	< 2 μg/g	10 μg/g
Carbamate insecticides	Inhibition of ChE activity in plasma		−50%
	in whole blood		−30%
	in red cells		−30%
Carbon disulphide	Iodine-azide test		6.5 (Vasak index)
Carbon monoxide	Carboxyhaemoglobin	< 1%	5% (non smokers)
Chromium (soluble compounds)	Urinary concentration	< 5 μg/g	30 μg/g
Cyclohexane	Exhaled air concentration	Nil	200 ppm
	Blood cyclohexanol	Nil	40 μg/dl
	Urinary cyclohexanol	Nil	3 mg/g
Dieldrin	Blood concentration	Nil	15 μg/dl
DNOC	Blood concentration	Nil	1 mg/dl
Endrin	Blood concentration	Nil	5 μg/dl
Ethylbenzene	Blood concentration	Nil	0.15 mg/dl
	Urinary mandelic acid		2g/g
Fluoride	Urinary concentration	< 0.4 mg/g	4 mg/g preshift 7 mg/g postshift
n-Hexane	Blood concentration	Nil	15 μg/dl
	Expired air concentration	Nil	50 ppm
	Urinary 2,5 hexanol	Nil	0.2 mg/g
	Urinary 2,5 hexanedione	Nil	5.5 mg/g
Halothane	Blood trifluoroacetic acid concentration	Nil	0.25 mg/dl
	Urinary trifluoracetic acid concentration	Nil	10 mg/g
Hexachlorobenzene	Blood concentration	Nil	0.3 mg/dl
Lead (inorganic)	Blood concentration	< 35 μg/dl	70 μg/dl
	Urinary concentration	< 50 μg/g	150 μg/g
	Urinary ALA	< 4.5 mg/g	10 mg/g
	Urinary Cp	< 100 μg/g	250 μg/g
	Free erythrocyte Protoporphyrin	< 75 μg/dl RBC	300 μg/dl RBC
	Zinc protoporphyrin	< 2.5 μg/g Hb	12.5 μg/g Hb

Chemical	Biological monitor	Normal value	Suggested Maximum
Lead (organic)	Urinary concentration	$< 50\ \mu g/g$	$150\ \mu g/g$
Mercury (inorganic)	Blood concentration	$< 2\ \mu g/dl$	$3\ \mu g/dl$
	Urinary concentration	$< 5\ \mu g/g$	$50\ \mu g/g$
Mercury, methyl	Blood concentration	$< 2\ \mu g/dl$	$10\ \mu g/dl$
Methanol	Urinary concentration	< 2.5 mg/g	7 mg/g
Methylene chloride	Blood concentration	Nil	$100\ \mu g/dl$
	Exhaled air concentration	Nil	35 ppm
	Carboxyhaemoglobin	$< 1\%$	5%
			(non smokers)
Methyl ethyl ketone	Urinary concentration	Nil	$2.5\ \mu g/g$
Nickel (soluble compounds)	Plasma concentration	$< 1\ \mu g/dl$	$1\ \mu g/dl$
	Urinary concentration	$< 5\ \mu g/g$	$70\ \mu g/g$
Nitrobenzene	Urinary p-aminophenol	Nil	5 mg/g
	Methaemoglobin	$< 2\%$	5%
Organophosphorus insecticides	Inhibition of ChE activity		
	in plasma		-50%
	in whole blood		-30%
	in red cells		-30%
Parathion	Urinary p-nitrophenol	Nil	2 mg/g
Pentachlorophenol	Urinary concentration	Nil	1 mg/g
Phenol	Urinary concentration	< 20 mg/g	300 mg/g
Selenium	Urinary concentration	$< 25\ \mu g/g$	$100\ \mu g/g$
Styrene	Urinary mandelic acid	< 5 mg/g	1 g/g
Tellurium	Urinary concentration	< 1 g/g	$1\ \mu g/g$
Tetrachloroethylene	Exhaled air concentration	Nil	4 ppm
Thallium	Urinary concentration	$< 1\ \mu g/g$	1 g/g
1,1,1-Trichloro-ethane	Exhaled air concentration	Nil	50 ppm
	Urinary trichloroethanol	Nil	30 mg/g
	Urinary trichloroethanol + trichloroacetic acid	Nil	50 mg/g
Toluene	Blood concentration	Nil	$100\ \mu g/dl$
	Exhaled air concentration	Nil	20 ppm
	Urinary hippuric acid	< 1.5 g/g	2.5 g/g
	Urinary o-cresol	< 0.3 mg/g	1 mg/g
Trichloroethylene	Blood concentration	Nil	0.6 mg/dl
	Exhaled air concentration	Nil	12 ppm
	Urinary trichloroethanol	Nil	125 mg/g
	Urinary trichloroacetic acid	Nil	75 mg/g
Vanadium	Urinary concentration	< 1 g/g	$50\ \mu g/g$
Vinyl chloride	Urinary thiodiglycolic acid	< 2 mg/g	2 mg/g
Xylene	Blood concentration	Nil	0.3 mg/dl
	Urinary methylhippuric acid	Nil	1.5 g/g

*All urinary concentrations in the Table are expressed per gram creatinine of biological monitoring is required. It may be sufficient to measure the concentration of the toxic substance (or a metabolite) in the blood or urine from which an index of the degree of absorption is obtained. On the other hand, it may be preferable to utilize a test which gives an indication of the degree of metabolic disturbance which is being produced by the absorbed material. In lead workers, for example, the blood or urine lead concentrations can be determined as measures of absorption whereas the concentrations of ALA in the urine or of protoporphyrin in the erythrocytes can be taken as indices of interference with haem synthesis. Similarly, the concentration of cadmium in the urine gives some guide to the amount of absorption, but the presence of proteinuria is the measure of the degree of interference with kidney tubular function. Exposure to physical hazards such as dust and noise is controlled by indirect methods which include radiography and pulmonary function tests for workers exposed to dusts and audiometry for men in noisy occupations.

Workers coming into contact with carcinogenic substances such as aromatic amines in the rubber industry or mineral oil in the engineering industry rely on periodical medical examinations to detect any premalignant change such as may be found, for example, in the skin of a man exposed to cutting oils. Where the changes are not visible, special techniques are employed, such as the examination of the urine of men in the rubber industry for malignant cells.

Some degree of prevention can also be achieved in certain occupations by pre-employment medical examinations. These not only establish a base line against which any future change can be judged but also allow unsuitable men to be disqualified from entering dangerous jobs. For example, one would not wish a chronic bronchitic to take up an occupation where there was a likelihood of exposure to dust or some other pulmonary irritant.

Biological thresholds

There is no legislation regulating the concentration of any toxic compound or its metabolites in blood, urine or exhaled air, but some recommended maxima are shown in Table 12.3.

Biological threshold values are based on the assumption that below some given concentration, toxic substances will not produce clinical poisoning even though there may be some degree of metabolic abnormality which is considered tolerable. The question which is constantly posed to those concerned with occupational health is, how much deviation from normal is *tolerable?*

In Russia and some of the other eastern European countries, threshold values have been established on the basis of behavioural studies with animals following the work of Pavlov. Animals are exposed to varying concentrations of the toxic substances under examination and its effects on conditioned reflex responses is noted. The levels permitted are just below those which at first produce alterations in behaviour. As shown in Table 12.4 these are generally much lower than levels permitted in this country. Studies on workers exposed to some heavy metals and solvents have reported abnormalities in behaviour as judged by their performance in a range of psychological tests and some changes in reproductive function are also said to occur in the absence of clinical signs or symptoms. There is no general agreement concerning the significance or validity of these results but nevertheless, their publication has led to a demand for a downward revision of present threshold values. Whether or not the results of the studies support such a move, it is important to remember that threshold values are not immutable but must constantly be revised in the light of new knowledge and of different expectations of those at work and of society at large.

On the basis of these results a number of authorities are pressing for a downward revision of present threshold values. Whether or not they are successful in their attempt, they have underlined the important principle that threshold values are not to be regarded as fixed and immutable, but must constantly be revised in the light of new knowledge.

NOTIFIABLE AND PRESCRIBED DISEASES

There are 16 industrial diseases which all doctors are required to notify to the Health and Safety Executive who publish periodic analyses of the number of cases by year (Table 12.5). Since the turn of the century, when the first diseases were notified, there has been a marked decline in the number of cases reported and in the number of fatalities. For example, in 1900 well over a thousand cases of lead poisoning with 38 fatalities were reported; nowadays well under 50 cases are notified each year and there has not been a case of industrial lead poisoning for many years. This trend towards fewer notifications reflects to a very large degree the improvement in working conditions which has taken place during this century. In well controlled modern industries with an effective occupational health service, the occupational physician would be surprised and disgraced if he were to see, for example, cases of metal

Table 12.4. Maximum allowable concentration of some harmful substances in various countries, in mg/m³*

Substance	United Kingdom (1972)	USA (1971–72)	Federal Republic of Germany (1971–72)	Switzerland (1971)	USSR (1970–71)	Czecho-slovakia (1970–71)	Poland (1970)
Acetone	2400	2400	2400	2400	200	800	200
Carbon dioxide	9000	9000	9000	9000	—	9000	—
Carbon monoxide	55	55	55	55	20	30	30
Lead	0.15	0.15	0.2	—	0.01	0.05	0.05
Methanol	260	260	260	260	5	100	50
Styrene	420	420	420	420	5	200	50
Toluene	375	375	750	380	50	200	100
Trichloroethylene	535	535	260	260	10	250	50
Xylene	435	435	870	435	50	200	100
Xylidine	25	25	25	25	3	5	—

*Data from various sources.

or solvent poisoning with any frequency. However, we should not be too complacent. One of the reasons for the small number of notifications is that many cases which do occur are unrecognized; it is hard to estimate the rate of under-reporting with any accuracy but it must be at least 50 per cent. Cases which occur will tend to do so in poorly controlled factories where there is unlikely to be any medical or nursing supervision and the onus will thus be on the general practitioner to make the diagnosis. Occupational medicine plays such an insignificant part in most undergraduate curricula that one should not be too critical of the fact that most general practitioners know little about the subject and so will not be adept at diagnosing occupational diseases. Should they do so, or should the diagnosis be made in hospital, it is likely that those concerned will be unaware that the disease must be notified. The probability of under-reporting is thus high.

Table 12.5. The notifiable diseases

Lead poisoning
Cadmium poisoning
Beryllium poisoning
Phosphorus poisoning
Manganese poisoning
Mercurial poisoning
Arsenic poisoning
Carbon disulphide poisoning
Aniline poisoning
Chronic benzene poisoning
Toxic jaundice
Toxic anaemia
Compressed air disease
Anthrax
Epitheliomatous ulceration
Chrome ulceration

The prescribed diseases are those which attract compensation from the Department of Health and Social Security. The Department has a standing Industrial Injuries Advisory Council which meets to make recommendations about the prescription of occupational diseases and in general their recommendations are accepted. The prescribed diseases include all those which are notifiable and 30 or so others. They tend to have a number of features in common. There are usually extremely stringent conditions which must have been met by the individual in terms of severity and length of exposure; the disability has usually to be great before attracting compensation; the disease is often rare and limited to a small group of workers and the amount of compensation is small. Amongst those diseases which have been recently prescribed are viral hepatitis, angiosarcoma of the liver and occupational deafness. One recently prescribed disease fails to meet most of the criteria which were referred to above; this is occupational asthma. Several causes of occupational asthma are prescribed and it has been estimated that many thousands of workers will be eligible for compensation; moreover it is likely that many new causes of the disease will be recognized which will attract compensation. The full list of prescribed diseases and the conditions under which workers may be eligible for compensation is published by the DHSS.

CENTRAL CONTROL

Governmental control of occupational health and safety was originally placed in the hands of the Factory Inspectorate which was established in 1833. The first Medical Inspector of Factories, Sir Thomas Legge, was not appointed until 1896 with the specific duty of reducing the dreadful toll of death and disease from lead and phosphorus poisoning. Other inspectorates have been established since then, all of whom came under the aegis of the Health and Safety Executive since the passage of the Health and Safety at Work Act in 1974. The inspectorates are responsible for the health and safety of all those who work (except for domestic servants, not a numerically significant cohort these days) in well over half a million establishments, factories and farms, mines and quarries and North Sea oil rigs. To accomplish this task there is provision for about a thousand inspectors; it takes only a few seconds on the calculator to see how frequently a work place may expect a routine visit from an inspector.

The medical arm of the Health and Safety Executive is the Employment Medical Advisory Service (EMAS) which operates on a regional basis and has provision for about 120 doctors; at the time of writing the service is about 50 per cent under-staffed. The duty of the Employment Medical Advisers is to give advice to anyone (medical or lay) on all matters to do with the effects of work on health or health on work. Again, the prospects of even a fully manned service of providing more than the most rudimentary health cover is obvious although it must be pointed out that many of the large industries have their own medical service. The chances of a factory with less than 100 employees having any medical cover, however, is less than 1 in 20 and only half the factories with more than 250 employees have a doctor; the majority of the work force of this country are employed in factories having fewer than 50 employees, and they are not likely to have any form of medical supervision whilst at work. Thus, there is a large potential target population for EMAS and again, it is clear that their facilities are much too limited to permit them to carry out their duties to the best effect.

Under the terms of the Health and Safety at Work Act, employers are obliged to ensure, so far as is reasonably practicable, the health, safety and welfare at work of all their employees. They must also ensure that plant and systems of work are safe and without risk to health, and that the working environment is without risk to health and provide such information, instruction, training and supervision as is necessary to ensure the health and safety of their work force. All those who manufacture or import materials must ensure that they are without risk to health if properly used. For their part, employees have a duty for their own health and safety and must co-operate with the employer so far as is necessary to fulfil that requirement. It is straining credulity to its limits to suppose that all employers—or indeed all employees—will obey the strictures of the Act without the sure and certain knowledge that any misdemeanours will be detected and punished. The Act can work effectively only if it is adequately enforced, and, as has been seen, the size of the Inspectorates and of EMAS is totally inadequate for the task and if these bodies are not considerably enlarged then some other form of control may be necessary.

There is one means by which effective local control of working conditions could be ensured; this is through the Safety Committees which the Health and Safety at Work Act requires to be set up at places of work. The members of the Safety Committees include representatives of the management and the Safety Representative appointed by the Trade Unions, and others who may be appointed *ex officio,* for instance the occupational nurse or physician, the occupational hygienist or the radiation protection officer. The Safety Representatives have wide ranging authority; they are entitled to inspect the work place and make recommendations to management, they are entitled to time off with pay in order to carry out their duties and they have a right to see the results of environmental monitoring. There is sometimes a fear in the minds of occupational physicians that the role of the safety representatives or the safety committee may conflict with their own, and there is no doubt that some safety representatives consider that the occupational physician is an ally of management rather than being an impartial adviser. With diplomacy and education, these difficulties can be overcome and the occupational physician can play an important role in feeding expert opinion into the safety committee and so help to improve local working conditions. The Safety Committee is potentially an important tool in controlling hazards at work and there seems to be no reason why it should not negotiate local exposure limits or local biological thresholds; it seems perfectly proper that those who are exposed to dangerous substances at work should have a large say in the extent to which they are prepared to take risks to their health providing that their views are based on sound toxicological or medical advice. The occupational physician should have nothing to fear from such an approach; his special expertise is required in order that the committee can function most satisfactorily and, in any case, all parties are ostensibly working towards the same end, that is to make the workplace as safe as it can possibly be.

CHAPTER 13/THE EFFECTS OF
WORK ON HEALTH

Although those who practice occupational medicine are principally concerned with the effects of work on health, they also have the important task of studying the effects which health may have on work; as the workplace becomes less dangerous and the prevalence of occupational disease decreases, this aspect of occupational medicine will assume greater importance. There are few medical conditions which are an absolute bar to work, but many may impair an individual's capacity to perform certain jobs to some degree and so a large part of the occupational physician's time is taken up in ensuring that the worker and his job are as well suited as possible. This process begins by assessing the health and capabilities of prospective employees before they are appointed. However, this does not mean to say that all new employees must necessarily be medically examined and indeed this is generally a poor use of the physician's time since the pick-up rate of abnormalities is likely to be small and by no means all those who attend for pre-employment medicals will be offered a job, nor will they all accept even if one is offered them. Nevertheless, they should all be subjected to some form of screening process and this can satisfactorily be undertaken by a trained occupational nurse who will ask each prospective employee to complete a health questionnaire which has been devised by the company doctor. The precise form which the questionnaire takes will depend upon individual preferences and special local requirements, but normally such a form is simple to construct and quick to administer. In the majority of cases the questionnaire will confirm that the worker is fit and no further action need be taken, except to inform the personnel department that there are no evident medical grounds for refusing the man work. A few questionnaires will need to be referred to the doctor for his opinion when there is some doubt as to the man's fitness to work, and some physicians may wish to check all the questionnaires themselves.

Whilst this simple screening procedure will generally be sufficient there will clearly be some categories of new employee who must be seen by the doctor. Those being taken on to work in a job which entails exposure to specific hazards, heavy metals, radiation or noise, for example, will need to be examined in order to establish base line clinical data which may need to be supplemented by laboratory investigations such as a blood lead estimation, full blood count or an audiogram. Food handlers must be free of gastro-intestinal infection and those who are to work in dialysis units must be hepatitis B antigen negative. Common sense dictates that men who are likely to be called upon to lift heavy loads must be free from a history of back pain, that lorry drivers or crane drivers must have good vision and no restriction of their visual fields, that those to be exposed to dust are free from lung disease, and so on. Each firm should be able to construct its own list of 'high risk' occupations which will require the special attention of the medical adviser.

Ill health which develops when the worker is in employment may require the doctor to re-assess his fitness to continue in his present job. The occupational physician is often asked to undertake this assessment by the management, especially if the worker in question is requiring frequent sickness absence. This is a perfectly reasonable request and should raise no problems of medical confidentiality so long as the doctor reports in general terms and does not enter into clinical details in his report to management without the written consent of the worker concerned. To assess fully fitness to work, the occupational physician may require more clinical information than is available to him from his own records and he may wish to supplement his knowledge of the case by writing to the general practitioner or a hospital consultant. Again, this should pose no ethical problems so long as consent is obtained from the worker and he is assured that any information which is forthcoming will remain confidential to the medical department.

In many firms all employees who are sick for a period of more than a few days or who have had a particularly severe illness are required to have a medical examination before their return to work. In some cases this is also done to encourage a man back to work after what seems an unseemly delay! The doctor should ensure that those who return from an illness are not put into situations with which they will be unable to cope, and that their return to work is supervised and graded as required. In many cases the return to work will be achieved most satisfactorily if there is a close liaison between the worker's general practitioner and the occupational physician, but all too often lines of communication between the two are poor and each chooses to operate without reference to the other, sometimes to the detriment of their patient.

Case indexes

In any firm there will be a proportion of men and women with non-occupational diseases of one sort or another, some serious, some trivial. Whether the physician tries to maintain a separate case index for a large number of diseases will depend upon his inclinations and his resources. Some diseases, however, should be given special attention, the most important of which are epilepsy and diabetes mellitus.

With proper medical supervision workers with epilepsy may undertake most jobs, and may drive so long as they have been without a fit for 3 years whilst awake regardless of whether or not they are receiving treatment Most doctors tend to be cautious in their dealings with epileptics, however, and prefer to keep them away from jobs which might involve contact with moving machinery or heights; many firms would also not allow them to drive. A *grand mal* fit is a spectacular and also a rather frightening episode for the layman to witness, and on this account alone epileptics are often not well tolerated by their work mates and so encouragement and support from the doctor is essential. A regular visit to the surgery will allow the doctor to satisfy himself that the man is taking his anticonvulsant therapy and it is prudent to keep in a small stock of anticonvulsants in case the man forgets to bring his own supply with him.

Diabetics in industry do not require the same degree of medical supervision as epileptics, but they need to be known so that they may be dealt with promptly and efficiently in an emergency. The most likely event is a hypoglycaemic coma and there should be provision for urine testing in the medical department and ideally a simple method for blood sugar estimation (such as the Ames Dextrostix). There should be no difficulty in distinguishing between hypoglycaemia and a diabetic coma; the latter is not a condition amenable to treatment in any setting other than a hospital, but the doctor should see that 50 per cent dextrose is available for the initial treatment of the former before the patient is referred elsewhere. It is also a sensible precaution to keep in a small supply of antidiabetic drugs for those who come to work without their own.

Psychiatric illness

Neurotic disorders are a common contribution to illness of all kinds and may often masquerade as physical disease. Estimates of the number of people with some kind of neurotic illness vary widely, but it has been suggested that they may represent 40 per cent of all general practitioner consultations. This must be reflected in the industrial setting and it has been estimated that the total number of days lost due to incapacity from 'nervous debility and headache' are rising, and are currently running at over 5 million a year. In addition to this, it is likely that between 20–25 per cent of all absenteeism can be attributed to neurosis.

In general terms, it is obvious that problems of adjustment and coping will be intimately related to productivity and efficiency in the industrial setting. There is evidence that the increase in the size of companies and in automation are producing effects on the motivation of individual workers and on his sense of identity with and responsibility to the company, and that he is not encouraged to see his individual importance to the firm as a whole. It is reasonable to suppose that this sense of alienation may have a greater effect on the more vulnerable personality and help to tip the balance between being able to cope, and not able to cope with work.

In more specific terms, one of the most important responsibilities of the occupational physician in the area of psychiatric illness is to identify those who are not declaring their symptoms. This is a serious consideration in those who have repeated sickness absence for apparently trivial conditions especially after promotion or an increase in responsibilities or whose efficiency and concentration are declining for no apparent reason. There are times when a change of job may be appropriate to alleviate a specific stress such as a personality clash with a supervisor, although it must always be borne in mind that the expressed cause of anxiety and depression may not reflect the true conflict which may be areas of the patient's life inaccessible to the intervention of the occupational physician. A common cause of failure to cope with work is a mismatch of the demands of the job and the worker's ability and it must be remembered that difficulties may arise equally because a man is doing a job beneath his capacity as well as when it is beyond him.

Other factors which may be predictive of the onset of psychiatric illness include an excess of zeal or over-conscientiousness in a worker who is attempting to make up for a fall in efficiency. Emotional or aggressive outbursts as a response to minor provocation in a previously stable worker should be taken seriously and the worker referred for psychiatric advice if it seems appropriate. Numerically, most illnesses of psychiatric origin in the work setting will be neurotic, but the possibility of psychotic breakdown must be considered if bizarre behaviour is reported.

The return to work after a psychiatric breakdown is complicated by two factors. Firstly, whatever the nature of the illness, a severe blow to the patient's self confidence has almost always occurred, and as a consequence he may undervalue his capacity and be unrealistically anxious about his ability to cope in future. Secondly, psychiatric illness still carries a stigma and not infrequently provokes fear and ridicule in others so that the reaction of close associates at work may have to be borne in mind. If it can be arranged it is often extremely helpful to grade the return to work in terms of time and responsibility, starting with a return of as little as one day a week with a steady increase unil the full working week is achieved. Ideally the degree of support required should be estimated for each individual; it can be harmful to be too protective and liaison between industry and the psychiatrist concerned can be very helpful in handling the return to work. The Disablement Resettlement Officer may also usefully be involved in these decisions (see below).

Workers who suffer from psychotic disorders pose particular problems. Many chronic schizophrenics are able to work in open industry, perhaps as part of the quota of jobs kept for the registered disabled, but they may be peculiarly susceptible to small changes in the job itself or to their immediate environment. Although they may work steadily and accurately, they are likely to work more slowly than the fit worker and so they should not usually be placed in situations where their workmates' output depends on theirs. If it is possible, tolerance of sickness absence should be exercised; the ability to work is crucial to the mental health of the schizophrenic and so it is preferable that they keep their jobs.

It must be remembered that whilst schizophrenia can be a disease which renders the patient less able and skilled after recurrences, manic-depressive psychosis is not. Most manic-depressives are perfectly able to continue their jobs at their previous level after attacks of illness and their return to this level must be facilitated whenever possible.

Finally, many psychotic patients need to return comparatively frequently to the clinic for long acting antipsychotic medication and for routine examinations, estimating serum lithium concentrations for example, and this should be actively encouraged by the industrial physician.

Alcoholism

Dependent drinking, or drinking to a degree which regularly impairs abilities in social, family or work relationships is the most important psychiatric problem in industry. This is not only due to the numbers affected but also because alcoholics conceal their condition either from a sense of shame or by denying that they have a problem. The heavy, non-dependent drinker has considerable nuisance value if he is drunk at work or hungover in bed on a Monday morning, but these activities do not pose the same problem to the occupational physician as the recognition and treatment of dependent drinking with its progressive mental and physical damage.

It is impossible to give a clear estimate of the prevalence of alcoholism, but one more reliable estimate is that there are 70,000 long-standing and 200,000 early alcoholics in England and Wales, making a prevalence of 8.5 per 1000 for the population at risk. The rate is likely to be higher than this in industry since the population at risk is comprised largely of those at work. The contribution made by the unemployed population, whilst not high in absolute terms is unknown. Although alcoholism in women and in the young is on the increase, the most susceptible group in industry remains the middle-aged man in his fifth decade, perhaps because the increase of female alcoholics is confined largely to the group of comparatively well off, non-employed housewives.

Recent drives to increase awareness of alcoholism in industry have had moderate success but the recognition of individuals who have become dependent upon alcohol is still inadequate. One should not have to wait until a man is suddenly found to have been admitted to an alcoholism unit, or until he has a withdrawal fit or patches of complete amnesia for events at work before the diagnosis is made. Deterioration to this degree places work colleagues at risk as well as the dependent drinker himself. There are many pointers towards the development of alcoholism which, taken together should provide enough suspicion for the physician to intervene. These include, persistent bad timekeeping, especially after weekends, and prolonged lunch hours. Withdrawal tremor may be marked early on in the working day or if an unusually long meeting prevents the worker from abolishing it by topping up with alcohol. Frequent absence due to 'gastritis' may also be significant especially if coupled with a decline in the standard of work and in moodiness. The carrying of alcohol on the person (except perhaps at Christmas) should immediately make one suspect dependence on alcohol.

The group which is perhaps most at risk of escaping detection is higher management; it is much easier to drink continuously during the day when alcohol is provided freely for refreshment and entertainment in the board room. Alcoholism is most prevalent in the highest and lowest social classes so company executives are greatly at risk, perhaps as a response to stress, and are encouraged by having alcohol readily available at work. The occupational physician should not shrink from his duty to protect and advise his colleagues in management despite the fact that he will be more tempted to accept the rationalizations of those who deny it is a problem whilst at the same time pointing to colleagues who apparently drink more than they do themselves. If alcoholism is suspected, the doctor should insist on the necessity for treatment which may involve psychiatric referral, or contact with Alcoholics Anonymous, or some other organization. For most alcoholics, continued abstinence is the index of successful treatment, although in some centres controlled drinking programmes have met with some success. It may therefore be seen as part of the occupational physician's duties to encourage the acceptance of abstinence in those at risk, and certainly a known interest in, and non-pejorative view of dependent drinking is likely to result in more open discussion and a more frank acknowledgement of the problem.

Treatment of alcoholics is rarely totally successful, at least in the early stages, and it must be remembered that the risk of recurrence is high, and the occupational physician should not consider that his job has been completed after the initial referral. Those who use alcohol as an anxiolytic are particularly at risk of becoming dependent and so there may be a case for recommending a change of job to one which is less stressful.

Finally, it is well to remember that the absence of drunkenness is no guide to the presence of alcoholism.

The disabled

Firms over a certain size are required to keep 3 per cent of their vacancies for the registered disabled but few comply with this regulation, especially in times of high unemployment. The tasks which a disabled person can perform will necessarily depend upon the nature of his disability but by no means all are restricted to minor clerical jobs or to answering the telephone.

The responsibility for training disabled persons, for finding them suitable employment and for maintaining the registers of disabled persons lies with the Disablement Resettlement Officer (DRO) and the Blind Persons' Resettlement Officer (BPRO). Both the DRO and BPRO are employed by the Employment Service Agency (ESA) which is one of the executive arms of the Manpower Services Commission (MSC) established in 1974. The ESA runs a number of Employment

Rehabilitation Centres at which disabled persons may attend for re-training or for a re-assessment of their capacity to work.

Some larger firms have their own rehabilitation centres which they encourage employers who have suffered accidents or severe illnesses to attend but not all will choose to do so.

Some disabled persons benefit from training schemes which are organized by the Training Services Agency of the MSC at their Skill-centres or technical colleges. These courses are intensive and usually last for about six months and may be supplemented by further periods of training when in employment.

Here, as in many other areas of occupational medicine, the patient is best served if there is a close working relationship between all with responsibilities towards him. In this case, there is a need for liaison between the occupational health services, the personnel at the Employment Rehabilitation Centres and Skillcentres, hospital staff and the general practitioner, but such liaison is often not well developed to put it mildly.

CHAPTER 14/OCCUPATIONAL
HEALTH SERVICES

The provision of health care for people at work varies enormously from industry to industry as may be seen in Table 14.1. From Table 14.2 it will be noted that a large proportion of the work force, most of whom work in factories employing less than 250 persons, has neither medical nor nursing cover. In general, where facilities are available the quality of the occupational health service is directly related to size. Thus, some of the largest private firms have sophisticated medical departments which employ a number of doctors and nurses, have surgeries at different points throughout the factory, provide rehabilitation, physiotherapy, laboratory and radiographic services, employ hygienists with the necessary back-up to undertake environmental surveys, and offer dental and other ancillary services free or on greatly subsidized terms. At the lower end of the scale are the large number of (usually small) firms who offer no kind of service at all beyond the provision of first aid facilities which all employers are obliged by law to provide in relation to the size of their work force. Since the most unhygienic working conditions are usually to be found in small factories, it follows that those most at risk have the least provision made for their health and safety.

Intermediate between these two extremes is an almost infinite variety of service, some run by full-time physicians, others by nurses with the supervision of part-time medical advisers, still others by nurses working with no direct medical help.

The nationalized industries are required to provide a comprehensive health service for their employees and theirs are undoubtedly amongst the best in the country. Ironically, the National Health Service, which is one of the largest of all the nationalized industries has only lately developed an awareness that it should have a health service for its own employees, largely in response to the recommendations contained within the Tonbridge report. The number of health service districts which have an effective occupational health service, however, is relatively small and the prospects for change are not great especially as there is no proper provision for the training of occupational physicians within the NHS. The DHSS has a duty to provide training posts for doctors in all specialties but it has established none for occupational physicians.

There has been a general agreement since the Dale Committee reported in 1951 that

> it is desirable that there should eventually be some comprehensive provision for occupational health covering not only industrial establishments of all kinds, both large and small, but also the non-industrial occupations . . .

Table 14.1. Provision of types of occupational health service by size of firm
% of firms

Number of employees	Medical and nursing staff	Medical staff only	Nursing staff only	Doctor on call only	Other staff only*	No service†	Total
0–10	0.8	0.4	0.4	0.4	0.0	98.0	100.0
11–24	1.2	0.5	0.4	3.8	0.9	93.2	100.0
25–49	0.9	1.5	1.5	7.1	2.4	86.6	100.0
50–99	0.9	4.1	2.2	8.4	4.4	80.0	100.0
100–249	5.4	9.8	4.9	11.0	2.6	66.3	100.0
250–499	22.5	9.8	14.9	7.1	6.3	39.4	100.0
500–999	42.9	11.1	21.0	6.3	3.2	15.5	100.0
1000–2499	78.9	4.4	7.0	3.8	0.6	5.3	100.0
2500–4999	80.0	2.5	7.5	2.5	0.0	7.5	100.0
5000+	76.9	3.8	7.6	7.7	0.0	4.0	100.0

*e.g. first aiders employed as such for at least 10 hours a week.
†Other then first aiders employed as such for less than 10 hours a week.
Reproduced with permission from *Occupational Health Services*, HMSO, 1977.

By contrast, there is no consensus on the means by which an occupational health service can be provided for the many smaller firms which have none at present. Governments of various shades have been urged by several medical bodies, including most notably the British Medical Association, to provide something akin to a National Occupational Health Service. Such an approach seems to me to be the only satisfactory solution. At present, occupational physicians are the only group of doctors not employed by the DHSS and, amongst other things, this has a markedly adverse effect on their training. If a national occupational health service were to be established in parallel with the NHS, not only would the imputation that occupational physicians are not entirely impartial disappear—no-one suggests that a cardiologist or a neurologist is a tool of *his* management (the DHSS)—but there would be an immediate benefit from improved contacts with other specialists in the NHS and better access to diagnostic and treatment facilities. Unfortunately, since the DHSS has only a minimal interest in preventive medicine, the chances that large sums of money will be deflected into creating an effective nationwide occupational health service are remote; this should not prevent interested parties from agitating for change and improvement, however.

Some firms which have no facilities of their own make some provision for their occupational health needs by subscribing to the 7 or 8 group occupational health services which there are in the United Kingdom, but the total number of workers who are covered in this way is relatively small.

Table 14.2. Frequency distribution of types of service, adjusted for sampling bias

Type of service	% firms	% workforce
Full-time medical and full-time nursing staff	0.5	16.5
Full-time medical and part-time nursing staff	0.1	0.1
Full-time medical staff; no nursing staff	0.04	0.3
Part-time medical and full-time nursing staff	1.5	25.2
Part-time medical and part-time nursing staff	0.4	2.4
Part-time medical staff; no nursing staff	1.1	5.1
Doctor on call; no nursing staff	6.8	6.1
Full-time nursing staff; no medical staff*	1.1	6.7
Part-time nursing staff; no medical staff*	0.9	1.6
No medical or nursing staff, but some other occupational health staff (e.g. first-aider employed as such for at least 10 hours a week)	2.7	1.8
No service except first-aiders employed as such for less than 10 hours a week	84.9	34.2
	100.0	100.0

*Other than a doctor on call.
Reproduced with permission from *Occupational Health Services*, HMSO, 1977.

The purposes of an occupational health service

The purpose of an occupational health service is to ensure that the health of men and women at work is not adversely affected by their occupation. The first duty of any occupational physician or occupational nurse must be towards securing that end. This principle is enshrined in Recommendation 112 of the International Labour Organization, formulated in 1959. This recommendation states that an occupational health service has the functions of:

1   protecting the worker against any health hazard which may arise out of their work or the conditions in which it is carried on;

2   contributing towards the workers' physical and mental adjustment, in particular, by the application of the work to the workers and their assignment to jobs for which they are suited; and

3   contributing to the establishment and maintenance of the highest degree of physical and mental well-being of the workers. In this country, most occupational health services concentrate their efforts in three main areas: prevention, adjustment to work, and treatment. The emphasis given to each varies from industry to industry as would be expected. In addition, one should not forget the research which is undertaken by doctors and others working in occupational health services and upon which the future development of the specialty largely depends.

Prevention

The prevention of occupationally induced diseases is paramount to the work of an occupational health service and involves not only protecting against well-recognized hazards but also the identification and evaluation of new hazards to health. This increasingly requires some form of epidemiological study, perhaps involving co-operation between different firms and collaboration with academic departments which have the necessary epidemiological and statistical skills to enable such a study to be carried out successfully. In the past occupational physicians and nurses have received little in the way of training in epidemiology but this deficiency is slowly becoming remedied, and future training programmes are certain to place more emphasis on this subject.

Programmes for preventing ill health in industry must, of course, contain a large educative component if they are to be successful. However, there is still too little effort given to the study of the best means whereby workers can be made aware of the potential hazards to which their job exposes them and of the steps which they can take themselves to protect their health. Likewise, management are not always made aware of their responsibilities in the preventive field as they ought to be, and it is the duty of occupational physicans and nurses to see that both sides of industry are better educated in these matters.

There is, of course, no reason why an occupational health service should restrict its health education solely to ocupational disease; it can, with advantage give advice on such matters as smoking and health, and on dietary habits, and can also make arrangements for services such as cervical cytology or mass radiography to be carried out within the work place.

Adjustment to work

This has been discussed in the previous chapter and will not be gone into further here.

Treatment

Occupational services do not normally offer a comprehensive treatment service except for accidents which may occur at work. Some firms will be able to offer nothing more than simple first-aid measures, but in the best case the occupational health service is equipped with a full range of resuscitation apparatus and may also have its own ambulance to ensure that accident victims are transported to hospital with the minimum delay.

The occupational health service will usually choose to undertake casualty-type work, the removal of foreign bodies from eyes, dressing of wounds, removal of sutures and so on, but it should not provide initial treatment for medical conditions since this properly falls within the province of the general practitioner or the hospital consultant.

Confidentiality

The physician in industry is sometimes in the invidious position of being viewed with mistrust by the employees because he is thought to be a tool of management, whilst management may think that he is not nearly obliging enough! If the occupational health service is to function well the doctor has to be seen to be impartial. Moreover the patients who attend the surgery must have confidence in the staff and must be assured that the doctor–patient (or nurse–patient) relationship is the same in the setting of the work place as elsewhere. Thus confidentiality must be respected and it must be made very clear to management that the medical records belong to the medical department and not the firm and that no one has the right of access to records by virtue of his position within the company.

The doctor in industry frequently encounters difficulties in trying to exercise his impartiality, however. For example, he may learn that a patient has a condition which may make him unfit for work, or worse, a potential danger were he to carry on, and the patient requests that management are not informed. The doctor will of course encourage the patient to change his job or seek medical treatment, or both, but if he is unsuccessful then he will have to tell the patient that his duty extends also to the other employees and to the management and that he cannot allow the patient to continue at work. If such a decision is transmitted to management, then it must be couched in general terms and no clinical details should be included.

On the other hand, the physician may also discover instances in which the health of workers has suffered as a direct conseqence of their work and he then has the duty to advise the men affected of their statutory benefits, if they are suffering from one of the prescribed diseases, and he should also discuss frankly with them the question of compensation if he considers management to be in any way culpable. If there is no possibility of compensation, he should nevertheless see that the men are treated as generously as possible by the company.

Perhaps the most important function of the occupational physician, however, is to ensure that all those who have a part to play in creating the safest possible working environment do so in harmony; disease is no respecter of class or political divisions, and progress will be achieved by co-operation and not conflict.

Future developments

As a society becomes more affluent its expectations increase and it will not tolerate those conditions under which its forefathers lived and worked. During the present century and especially in the last 3 decades, working conditions for the majority of people have improved enormously. This has been due not only to the introduction of better control of hazards at the work place and to improved medical supervision but also to the change in the pattern of industry in the country. Many of the traditional heavy industries have contracted or disappeared altogether and a much greater proportion of the work force is employed in service industries or in light industry in which the risks to health are relatively small. No occupational physician who practices in the developed countries in the future will have personal experience of the huge numbers of cases of toxic diseases which are so elegantly described in Donald Hunter's *Diseases of Occupations.* Hunter was able to conduct ward rounds at the London Hospital in the late 1940s during which he could demonstrate a seemingly endless number of cases such as lead poisoning, mercury poisoning, toxic jaundice or silicosis, cases which formed the basis of his book, for he never was employed in industry. Today the book is read more as an important social document than as a medical text since Hunter's medical practice is beyond our experience in the same way that cholera and smallpox no longer form a part of the day to day practice of a community physician.

The corollary of this decline in the prevalence of the classic occupational diseases is that those who work in the new conditions have new expectations. And the concerns of the present generation of workers are becoming increasingly centred around smaller deviations from normality, and around behavioural and reproductive effects of exposure to potentially toxic materials and about the possible mutagenic or carcinogenic risks at the workplace. The occupational physician has necessarily to adapt to this change; much of the research into the effects of work on health is now in the hands of epidemiologists rather than clinicians, dermatologists and chest physicians investigate occupational skin diseases and chest diseases and the control of accidents, through which most lives are lost at work, is the province of the safety officer. What is the occupational physician to do? He will first of all have to concentrate increasingly on the effects of health on work and he may also find that he becomes the source of general health education; if present economic trends continue, much of his time may also be spent in preparing people to spend the large part of their life out of work.

Occupational medicine in the fully developed countries therefore seems about to enter into a sub-clinical period, where opinion will be given in shades of grey rather than in black and white and where there is a danger that words will come to mean whatever the speaker wishes them to mean. On the broader front, however, things are different. Occupational health in many of the developing countries has many similarities to that in the UK in the 1920s and 30s and it is the duty of fully industrialized nations to share their experience with the developing countries in order that they do not repeat the mistakes which we made.

APPENDIX

Some threshold limit values—8 hour time weighted average values (TLV) and 10 minute TWA values for short term exposure limits (STEL)

Substance	TLV Parts/10^6	mg/m^3	STEL Parts/10^6	mg/m^3
Acetone	1000	2400	1250	3000
Acrylamide—skin*	—	0.3	—	0.6
Acrylonitrile—skin (control limit)	2	4	—	—
Aldrin—skin	—	0.25	—	0.75
Aluminium, metal and oxide	—	10	—	20
Ammonia	25	18	35	27
Aniline—skin	2	10	5	20
Antimony and compounds (as Sb)	—	0.5	—	—
Arsenic and compounds (as As)	—	0.2	—	—
Arsine	0.05	0.2	—	—
Azinphos-methyl—skin	—	0.2	—	0.6
Barium (soluble compounds)	—	0.5	—	—
Benzene—skin	10	30	—	—
Beryllium	—	0.002	—	—
Bromine	0.1	0.7	0.3	2
Cadmium, dusts and salts (as Cd)	—	0.05	—	0.2
Cadmium oxide fume (as Cd)	—	0.05	—	0.05
Calcium oxide	—	2	—	—
Carbon black	—	3.5	—	7
Carbon dioxide	5000	9000	15 000	27 000
Carbon disulphide—skin (control limit)	10	30	—	—
Carbon monoxide	50	55	400	440
Carbon tetrachloride—skin	10	65	20	130
Chlorine	1	3	3	9
Chlorobenzene	75	350	—	—

*The word 'skin' denotes the fact that a significant amount of the material may be absorbed through the skin and mucous membranes.

Substance	TLV Parts/10^6	mg/m^3	STEL Parts/10^6	mg/m^3
Chlorinated biphenyls—skin				
(42 per cent chlorine)	—	1	—	2
(54 per cent chlorine)	—	0.5	—	1
Chloroform	10	50	—	—
Chromium	—	0.5	—	—
Chromium (II) compounds				
(as Cr)	—	0.5	—	—
Chromium (III) compounds				
(as Cr)	—	0.5	—	—
Chromium (VI) compounds				
(as Cr)	—	0.05	—	—
Coal dust, containing				
< 5 per cent respirable quartz	—	2	—	—
> 5 per cent respirable quartz	See section on airborne dusts			
Coal dust in mines				
(control limit)	—	7	—	—
Cobalt and compounds (as Co)	—	0.1	—	—
Copper fume	—	0.2	—	—
Dusts and mists	—	1	—	2
Cotton dust (total dust				
less fly)	—	0.5	—	—
Cresol, all isomers—skin	5	22	—	—
Cristabolite				
(total dust)	—	0.15	—	—
Cyanide, as CN—skin	—	5	—	—
Cyclohexane	300	1050	375	1300
DDT	—	1	—	3
Demeton—skin	0.01	0.1	0.03	0.3
1,2-Dichlorobenzene	50	300	50	300
1,4-Dichlorobenzene	75	450	110	675
1,2-Dichloroethane	10	40	15	60
Dichlorovos—skin	0.1	1	0.3	3
Dieldrin—skin	—	0.25	—	0.75
Diisobutyl ketone	25	150	—	—
Dinitrobenzene (all isomers)—				
skin	0.15	1	0.5	3
Dinitro-o-cresol—skin	—	0.2	—	0.6
Dinitrotoluene—skin	—	1.5	—	5
Dioxan (diethylene dioxide)—				
skin	50	—	—	—
Diphenylamine	—	10	—	20
Diquat	—	0.5	—	1
Endrin—skin	—	0.1	—	0.3
Epichlorhydrin—skin	5	20	10	40

Substance	TLV Parts/10^6	mg/m^3	STEL Parts/10^6	mg/m^3
Ethyl alcohol	1000	1900	—	—
Ethyl ether	400	1200	500	1500
Ethylene chlorohydrin—skin	1	3	1	3
Ethylene dinitrate—skin	0.2	2	0.2	2
Ethylene glycol monobutyl ether—skin	50	240	150	720
Ethylene glycol monoethyl ether—skin	100	370	150	560
Ethylene glycol monomethyl ether—skin	25	80	35	120
Ethylene glycol particulate	—	10	—	20
vapour	100	250	125	325
Fluoride (as F)	—	2.5	—	—
Fluorine	1	2	2	4
Formaldehyde	2	3	2	3
Formic acid	5	9	—	—
Furfural—skin	5	20	15	60
Glutaraldehyde	0.2	0.7	0.2	0.7
Glycerol trinitrate—skin	0.2	2	0.2	2
Graphite (synthetic)	—	10	—	—
Heptachlor—skin	—	0.5	—	2
n—Hexane	100	360	125	450
Hydrogen bromide	3	10	—	—
Hydrogen chloride	5	7	5	7
Hydrogen cyanide—skin	10	10	10	10
Hydrogen fluoride (as F)	3	2.5	6	5
Hydrogen peroxide	1	1.5	2	3
Hydrogen sulphide	10	14	15	21
Hydroquinone	—	2	—	4
Iodine	0.1	1	0.1	1
Iron oxide fume (as Fe)	—	5	—	10
Iron salts, soluble (as Fe)	—	1	—	2
Isocyantes, all (as NCO) (control limit)	—	0.02	—	0.07
Isophorone	2	25	2	25
Lead, all componds except for tetraethyl lead (control limit)	—	0.15	—	—
Limestone	—	10	—	20
Lindane—skin	—	0.5	—	1.5
Magnesium oxide fume	—	10	—	—
Malathion—skin	—	10	—	—
Manganese and compounds (as Mn)	—	5	—	5

Substance	TLV Parts/10^6	mg/m^3	STEL Parts/10^6	mg/m^3
Manganese fume (as Mn)	—	1	—	3
Mercury alkyls (as Hg) — skin	—	0.01	—	0.03
Mercury and compounds, except alkyls (as Hg)	—	0.05	—	0.15
Methanol — skin	200	260	250	310
Methyl alcohol — skin	200	260	250	325
Methyl bromide — skin	15	60	—	—
Methyl butyl ketone	25	100	40	165
Methyl chloride	100	210	125	260
Methylcyclopentadienyl manganese tricarbonyl (as Mn) — skin	0.1	0.2	0.3	0.6
Methyl demeton — skin	—	0.5	—	1.5
Methyl ethyl ketone	200	590	300	885
Methyl isobutyl ketone — skin	100	410	125	510
Methyl methacrylate — skin	10	35	—	—
Methyl parathion — skin	—	0.2	—	0.6
Methylene chloride	200	700	250	870
Mica				
total dust	—	10	—	—
respirable dust	—	1	—	—
Molybdenum (as Mo)				
soluble compounds	—	5	—	10
insoluble compounds	—	10	—	20
Naphthalene	10	50	15	75
Nickel carbonate (as Ni)	0.05	0.35	—	—
Nickel carbonyl	0.001	0.007	—	—
Nickel metal	—	1	—	—
Nickel, soluble compounds (as Ni)	—	0.1	—	0.3
Nitric acid	2	5	4	10
Nitric oxide	25	30	35	45
Nitrobenzene — skin	1	5	2	10
Nitrogen dioxide	5	9	5	9
Nitrotoluene — skin	5	30	10	60
Oil mist	—	5	—	10
Osmium tetroxide (as Os)	0.0002	0.002	0.0006	0.006
Ozone	0.1	0.2	0.3	0.6
Paraffin wax fume	—	2	—	6
Paraquat, respirable sizes	—	0.1	—	—
Parathion — skin	—	0.2	—	0.6
Perchloroethylene — skin	100	670	150	1000

Substance	TLV Parts/10^6	mg/m³	STEL Parts/10^6	mg/m³
Phenol—skin	5	19	10	38
Phenylhydrazine—skin	5	20	10	45
Phosdrin (Mevinphos)—skin	0.01	0.1	0.03	0.3
Phosgene (carbonyl chloride)	0.10	0.4	—	—
Phosphine	0.3	0.4	1	1
Phosphoric acid	—	1	—	3
Phosphorus (yellow)	—	0.1	—	0.3
Phosphorus pentachloride	0.1	1	—	—
Phosphorous trichloride	0.5	3	—	—
Phthalic anhydride	1	6	4	24
Platinum (soluble salts), (as Pt)	—	0.002	—	—
Polyvinyl chloride				
total dust	—	10	—	—
respirable dust	—	5	—	—
Potassium hydroxide	—	2	—	2
Propylene glycol dinitrate—				
skin	0.2	2	0.2	2
Propylene glycol monomethyl				
ether	100	360	150	540
Pyrethrins	—	5	—	10
Quartz, crystalline				
total dust	—	0.3	—	—
respirable dust	—	0.1	—	—
Quinone	0.1	0.4	0.3	1
Resin core solder pyrollysis				
products (as formaldehyde)	—	0.1	—	0.3
Selenium compounds (as Se)	—	0.2	—	—
Selenium hexafluoride (as Se)	0.05	0.2	—	—
Silica, amorphous				
total dust	—	0.3	—	—
respirable dust	—	0.1	—	—
Silver	—	0.1	—	—
Silver, soluble compounds				
(as Ag)	—	0.01	—	0.03
Sodium fluoroacetate—skin	—	0.05	—	0.15
Sodium hydroxide	—	2	—	2
Stibene	0.1	0.5	0.3	1.5
Styrene (control limit)	100	420	250	1050
Styrene monomer	100	420	125	525
Sulphur dioxide	2	5	5	13
2,4,5-T	—	10	—	20
Sulphuric acid	—	1	—	—
Talc				
total dust	—	10	—	—
respirable dust	—	1	—	—

Substance	TLV Parts/10^6	mg/m^3	STEL Parts/10^6	mg/m^3
Tantalum	—	5	—	10
Tellurium and compounds except hexafluoride (as Te)	—	0.1	—	—
Tellurium hexafluoride (as Te)	0.02	0.2	—	—
TEPP—skin	0.004	0.05	0.012	0.15
Tetrachloroethane—skin	5	35	10	70
Tetrachloroethylene	100	670	150	1000
Tetraethyl lead (as Pb)— skin (control limit)	—	0.10	—	—
Thallium, soluble compounds (as Tl)—skin	—	0.1	—	—
Tin, inorganic compounds (as Sn)	—	2	—	4
Tin, organic compounds (as Sn)	—	0.1	—	0.2
Titanium dioxide	—	10	—	20
Toluene—skin	100	375	150	560
Trichloroethylene—skin (control limit)	100	535	150	802
1,1,1-Trichloroethane	350	1900	450	2450
Trinitrotoluene	—	0.5	—	0.5
Triorthocresyl phosphate	—	0.1	—	0.3
Tungsten and compounds (as W) soluble		1	—	3
insoluble	—	5	—	10
Vanadium pentoxide (as V) dust	—	0.5	—	1.5
fume	—	0.05	—	0.05
Vinyl chloride monomer (control limit)	3 (averaged over 1 year)	—	—
	5 (averaged over 1 month)	—	—
	6 (averaged over 1 week)	—	—
	7 (averaged over 8 hours)	—	—
	8 (averaged over 1 hour)	—	—
Welding fume	—	5	—	—
White spirit	100	575	125	720
Wood dust (non-allergenic)	—	5	—	10
Xylene, all isomers—skin	100	435	150	650
Xylidine—skin	5	25	10	50
Zinc chloride fume	—	1	—	2
Zinc chromate (as Cr)	—	0.05	—	—
Zinc oxide fume	—	5	—	10
Zinc distearate	—	10	—	20

Dusts

Asbestos

Asbestos dust (control limit)	Fibres/ml
Dust consisting of or containing any crocidolite or amosite	0.2 when measured or calculated in relation to a 4-hour reference period
Dust consisting of or containing other types of asbestos but not crocidolite or amosite	0.5 when measured or calculated in relation to a 4-hour reference period

Airborne dusts

Mineral dusts containing silica. To calculate the recommended limits for mineral dusts containing crystalline silica, the following formulae should be used.

Total dust, respirable and non-respirable:

$$8 \text{ hr TWA (mg/m}^3) = \frac{30}{\% \text{ quartz} + 3}$$

Respirable dust only:

$$8 \text{ hr TWA (mg/m}^3) = \frac{10}{\% \text{ respirable quartz} + 2}$$

For mineral dusts which contain cristobalite or tridymite, a value equal to one half of that obtained from the above formulae should be used.

Coal dust. Permitted levels of respirable coal dust in coal mines are laid down in the Coal Mines (Respirable Dust) Regulations 1975 and the Coal Mines (Respirable Dust Amendment) Regulations 1978.

When exposure occurs to coal dust containing more than 5 per cent quartz in workplaces other than coal mines, the formulae for mineral dust containing crystalline silica should be used.

Graphite. For natural or synthetic graphite which contains more than 1 per cent quartz, the formulae for mineral dusts containing silica should be used.

FURTHER READING

Further information on the topics discussed here may be obtained from the following sources; this is by no means an exhaustive list.

Doull J., Klaassen C.D. and Amdur M.D. *Cassarett and Doull's Toxicology*, 2nd edn. Macmillan, 1980.

Fisher A.A. *Contact Dermatitis*, Lea and Febiger, 1973.

Hamilton A. and Hardy H.L. *Industrial Toxicology*, revised by A.J. Finkel. John Wright, 1983.

Hunter D. *The Diseases of Occupations*, 6th edn. Hodder and Stoughton, 1978.

International Labour Office, *Encyclopaedia of Occupational Health and Safety*, 3rd edn. 1983 (2 vols).

Parkes W.R. *Occupational Lung Disorders*, 2nd edn. Butterworth, 1982.

Rom W.N. *Environmental and Occupational Medicine*, Little, Brown & Co, 1983.

Schilling R.S.F. *Occupational Health Practice*, 2nd edn. Butterworth, 1981.

Searle C.E. *Chemical Carcinogens.* American Chemical Society, 1976.

Waldron H.A. and Harrington J.M *Occupational Hygiene*, Blackwell Scientific Publications, 1981.

Zenz C. *Developments in Occupational Medicine.* Year Book Medical Publishers, 1980.

INDEX

Index